Mechanisms of chemical carcinogenesis

Dedicated to my dear wife

Mechanisms of chemical carcinogenesis

D. E. Hathway, DSc, PhD(Lond), CBiol, FIBiol, FRCPath, CChem, FRSC
Fellow of the University of Durham

Formerly Company Research Associate, Imperial Chemical Industries;
and Visiting Reader (in Toxicology) of the University of Bradford

Butterworths
London Boston Durban Singapore Sydney Toronto Wellington

All rights reserved. No part of this publication may be reproduced or transmitted in any form or by any means including photocopying and recording, without the written permission of the copyright holder, application for which should be addressed to the publishers. Such written permission must also be obtained before any part of this publication is stored in a retrieval system of any nature.

This book is sold subject to the Standard Conditions of Sale of Net Books and may not be re-sold in the UK below the net price given by the Publishers in their current price list.

First published 1986

© Butterworth & Co (Publishers) Ltd, 1986

British Library Cataloguing in Publication Data

Hathway, D.E.
   Mechanisms of chemical carcinogenesis.
   1. Carcinogens   2. Chemicals—Physiological effect
   I. Title
   616.99′4071   RC268.6
ISBN 0–408–11570–X

Library of Congress Cataloging in Publication Data

Hathway, D.E.
   Mechanisms of chemical carcinogenesis.

   Includes bibliographies and index.
   1. Carcinogenesis.   2. Carcinogens—Metabolism
3. Chemicals—Physiological effect.   I. Title.
[DNLM: 1. Carcinogens.   2. Neoplasms—chemically induced.   QZ 202 H363m]
RC268.5.H38   1985   616.99′4071   85-18982
ISBN 0–408–11570–X

Typeset by Scribe Design, Gillingham, Kent
Printed in Great Britain at the University Press, Cambridge

Preface

My perception from a long period of research on outstanding problems of carcinogenicity and toxicity is that the cancer field tends to be fragmented. Whilst several subject areas, including the epidemiology, chemical carcinogenesis, the role of oncogenic viruses, tumour aetiology and pathogenesis, metastasis and cancer chemotherapy, are currently being intensively investigated, it is virtually impossible for a single worker to keep abreast of the progress that is being made in all of these specialisms. It was for this reason that I thought that I should like to write a book which would stress the fundamental mechanisms of chemical carcinogenesis. The points that will be raised and the scientific problems that will be discussed do not belong exclusively to this subject and are also relevant to some other branches of cancer science, such as cancer chemotherapy, epidemiological analysis and preventive medicine.

This book is not a textbook. It is intended to summarize the main experimental evidence and theory about this rapidly growing branch of science. In places, I have chosen certain examples from a mass of literature and doubtless neglected others of equal merit. The only alternative would have been to have filled several volumes. Nevertheless, there may be some advantage in trying to survey the interactions of chemical carcinogens with native DNA, the activation of normal cellular (nucleotide) sequences, and the transforming role of the activated genes in a short book. A bird's-eye view may gain in balance what it loses in precision. The book is timely, because of renewed interest in molecular genetics. In fact, recent advances at the genetic level concur with the resulting data from epidemiological analysis and the chemical/biochemical investigation of cellular transformation.

The subject matter of this book is organized into chapters that deal with separate subjects and, whilst this style exposes the relevant mechanisms, it inevitably incurs a slight reiteration about some carcinogens and contributing ideas, but any such overlapping material is treated from rather different points of view in the various contexts concerned.

I hope that the book will be useful, particularly to workers involved with cancer research, molecular biology and toxicology, as well as to specialists in drug development, industrial hygiene and occupational medicine.

I should like to express my gratitude for the stimulating conversation of my colleagues and friends, especially Drs. Peter O'Connor, Francis Roe, Frank Rose CBE FRS and Roy Saffhill and Professors Charles Evans FRS, Leon Golberg,

Peter Magee and Cesare Maltoni, and my indebtedness to the published work, including:

T. Boveri (1914) *Zur Frage der Entstehung maligner Tumoren*
K.H. Bauer (1928) *Mutationstheorie der Geschwulst-Entstehung*
J.B.S. Haldane (1954) *Biochemistry of Genetics*
A. Pullman and B. Pullman (1955) *Cancérisation par les substances chimiques et structure moléculaire*
Alexander Haddow (1959) P.F. Frankland Memorial Lecture, *Chemical Mechanisms in the Induction of Cancer*
James Miller (1970) G.H.A. Clowes Memorial Lecture, *Carcinogenesis by Chemicals: an Overview*.

The author would like to thank Miss Sue Deeley of Butterworth Scientific Limited for her professional help and interest, Dr I.F.H. Purchase and his colleagues of ICI's Central Toxicology Laboratory for their continuing support, the staff of the Bodleian, University of Oxford, and Mrs Marjory J. Purser for her invaluable and unstinting help in preparing the typescript.

D.E. Hathway

Abbreviations

A	adenosine
2AAF	*N*-(2-fluorenyl)acetamide
BCPN	*N*-*n*-butyl-*N*-(3-carboxypropyl)nitrosamine
BHA	a mixture of 2- and 3-*tert*-butyl-4-methoxyphenol
BHBN	*N*-*n*-butyl-*N*-(4-hydroxybutyl)nitrosamine
BHT	3,5-di-*tert*-butyl-4-hydroxytoluene
C	cytidine
dA	deoxyribosyladenine
DAB	4-dimethylamino-azobenzene
dAMP	deoxyribosyladenine 5'-phosphate
dC	deoxyribosylcytosine
dCMP	deoxyribosylcytosine 5'-phosphate
dCTP	deoxyribosylcytosine 5'-triphosphate
DEN	*N*,*N*-diethylnitrosamine
DES	diethyl sulphate
dG	deoxyribosylguanine
dGMP	deoxyribosylguanine 5'-phosphate
dGTP	deoxyribosylguanine 5'-triphosphate
DIC (DTIC)	5-(3,3-dimethyl-1-triazeno)imidazole-4-carboxamide
DMN	*N*,*N*-dimethylnitrosamine
DMPT	3,3-dimethyl-1-phenyltriazene
DMS	dimethyl sulphate
DNA	deoxyribonucleic acid
dT	thymidine
dTMP	thymidine 5'-phosphate
dTTP	thymidine 5'-triphosphate
EGF	epidermal growth factor or epidermal polypeptide hormone
EMS	ethyl methane sulphonate
ENNG	*N*-ethyl-*N'*-nitro-*N*-nitrosoguanidine
ENU	*N*-ethyl-*N*-nitrosourea
G	guanosine
MAB	*N*-4-methylamino-azobenzene
MMS	methyl methane sulphonate
MNNG	*N*-methyl-*N'*-nitro-*N*-nitrosoguanidine

MNU	*N*-methyl-*N*-nitrosourea
MPT	3-methyl-1-phenyltriazene
mRNA	messenger ribonucleic acid
NADPH	reduced nicotinamide adenine dinucleotide phosphate
PAPS	3′-phosphoadenosine-5′-phosphosulphate
PCBs	polychlorinated biphenyls
PDGF	platelet-derived growth factor
poly(dA-dT)	alternating copolymer of dA and dT
poly(dC-dG)	alternating copolymer of dC and dG
poly(dC-3-Me-dC)	alternating copolymer of dC and 3-Me-dC
poly(UG)	random copolymer of uridine and guanosine
RNA	ribonucleic acid
rRNA	ribosomal ribonucleic acid
S_N1, S_N2	reaction mechanisms, named by Ingold; S_N1 stands for substituting nucleophilic monomolecular
T	ribosylthymine
$t_{0.5}$	biological half-life, e.g. of a reactive carcinogen intermediate
TPA	12,*O*-tetradecanoylphorbol-13-acetate
tRNA	transfer ribonucleic acid
UDPGT	uridine 5′-pyrophosphate glucuronyl transferase

Contents

1 **Introduction**   1
  Landmarks in the recognition of chemical carcinogenesis   2
  Developing theory from its roots in experiment   7
  Bibliography and references   11

2 **Activation of chemical carcinogens in the mammal**   14
  Presumptive evidence of metabolic activation   14
  Reactive metabolites of chemical carcinogens   17
  Biosynthesis of reactive metabolites and matching tissue specificities   36
  Bibliography and references   41

3 **Authenticated interactions with nucleic acid**   47
  Aromatic amines and amino-azo dyes   47
  Nitrosamines and 3-alkyl-1-phenyltriazines   54
  Metals   56
  Vinyl chloride   56
  Glycidaldehyde   58
  Aflatoxins   60
  Polycyclic aromatic hydrocarbons   61
  Safrole   64
  Concluding remarks   64
  Bibliography and references   64

4 **Mechanisms in perspective: biological significance of modified deoxyribonucleoside residues in DNA**   67
  Repair of biochemical lesions in DNA   68
  Miscoding induced by carcinogens during directed nucleic acid biosynthesis   73
  Effects on the biosynthesis of inter-related macromolecules   79
  Bibliography and references   82

5 **Mechanisms in perspective: inhibition of tumour induction**   85
  Inhibition of tumour initiation by metabolic inducers and inhibitors   86
  Inhibition of tumour initiation by the interaction of nucleophiles with reactive carcinogen intermediates   92

    Inhibition of tumour initiation through the induction of DNA-repair mechanisms   95
    Bibliography and references   97

6   Mechanisms in perspective: tumour promotion   100
    Two-stage carcinogenesis in the skin system   101
    The croton oil promoters   102
    Tumour promoters for other physiological systems   104
    Other experimental models of two-stage carcinogenesis   105
    Mode of action of tumour promotion in the skin   107
    Bibliography and references   109

7   Standard mutational theory of cancer and the impact of contingent advances in genetics   113
    Somatic cell mutation   113
    Cancer models   115
    The 'oncogene'/proto-oncogene concept   118
    The developing 'oncogene' story   119
    Activation of 'oncogenes'   121
    Proteins encoded by activated 'oncogenes'   123
    Concluding remarks   124
    Bibliography and references   125

Index   129

Chapter 1
Introduction

Carcinogesis has to do with the mode of action and so-called causative mechanisms of tumour induction. The record of case histories of cancer spreads over more than two centuries, and knowledge derived from animal experiments extends over more than 70 years. Thus, it is salutary to realize that the present understanding of carcinogenesis has been hardly won.

Whilst all biological phenomena are complicated, if they are investigated in depth, the parameters involved in the transformation of normal cells into tumour cells seem to be more profound than those implicated in other disease processes, for example in inflammatory or degenerative disease processes. This becomes evident from consideration of the multitude of structurally dissimilar chemical carcinogens, and the members of physical agents and oncogenic viruses which can effect tumour induction, in marked contrast to the single aetiological factor that generally elicits a pathological change.

A state of knowledge has now been reached at which the complexity of the problem of how normal cells are transformed into tumour cells has been gauged, and the various contributive factors seem to have been appraised. Substantial progress has been made by different experimental approaches. Thus, considerable evidence has been obtained on the modification of DNA nucleoside residues by interaction with reactive carcinogen metabolites, on the biological significance of the resulting nucleoside analogues in the native DNA, and on the sort of mutagenicity which ensues. This approach links with direct mutagenicity testing in genetically manipulated bacterial strains. Another means of investigating the underlying biological mechanisms arises from the parallel that has been found between the transformation of normal cellular genes into 'oncogenes' by viral regulation and the activation of normal cellular (nucleotide) sequences through a redistribution of the genes, after significant modification of the DNA by chemical carcinogens. Thus, DNA-mediated gene-transfer methods facilitate the detection of dominant transforming genes, or 'oncogenes', and detailed analysis has elucidated the changes which took place in the activation process. This approach links with the sort of cell types which are transformable. The recent identification of an endogenous protein, with known physiological effects on normal cells, as the translational product of an authenticated 'oncogene' stresses the value of the genetic approach. This finding presages a role for dosimetry in the transformation of genes.

Accordingly, an analysis, at any rate an interim analysis, of all of the progress that has been made would seem to be timely, although the data resulting from disparate approaches has not been fully integrated. Moreover, according to some sources, cancer mortality in the human population appears to be increasing, even if allowance be made for an increasing population and increased life expectancy (Terry Report, 1964; Süss, Kinzel and Scribner, 1970; Meleka, 1983). This sweeping statement needs further qualification, however, as much of the apparent increase is due to smoking habits and, if mortality from lung cancer be excluded, then there is an overall decrease as, for example, gastrointestinal tract cancer is decreasing. Thus, whilst some cancers, like the lung ones, are increasing, others, like aromatic amine bladder cancer and benzene leukaemia (see below), are declining. A proper understanding of the mechanisms of chemical carcinogenesis is fundamental to the cancer problem and a prerequisite both of preventive hygiene and medicine and of cancer chemotherapy.

It might be appropriate at the start of this narrative to draw attention to some landmarks in our awareness of chemical carcinogenesis and to some historical milestones in the developing theory.

Landmarks in the recognition of chemical carcinogenesis

Aromatic amine bladder cancer

Rehn (1895) reported a correlation between exposure to aromatic amines and cancer, having discovered three men suffering from bladder cancer, who were engaged in making fuchsin from commercial aniline at the same chemical works in Basel. A fourth case had been employed on the same process at another works. Bladder cancer is sufficiently rare for a cluster of a few cases to be highly significant. Subsequently, the occurrence of this occupational disease was confirmed in every country with a manufacturing chemical industry; the causative agents included commercial aniline, 4-aminobiphenyl, benzidine and 2-naphthylamine.

In a study of 4622 British chemical workers, Case et al. (1954) found 262 cases of bladder cancer, including 34 cases of workers who had been exposed only to benzidine. As only 0.72 bladder cancer cases would be expected in a corresponding background population, the incidence of benzidine bladder cancer was highly significant. Supporting evidence for benzidine bladder cancer came from chemical works in France (Billiard-Duchesne, 1959) and the United States (Goldwater, Rosso and Kleinfeld, 1965; Mancuso and El-Attar, 1967) and from experiments in dogs (Spitz, Maguigan and Dobriner, 1950). It is not known whether the benzidine derivatives, dianisidine (3,3'-dimethoxybenzidine), 3,3'-dichlorobenzidine and o,o'-tolidine (2,2'-diamino-4,4'-dimethylbiphenyl), which were often made in the same chemical plant as benzidine, contributed to the human bladder tumours ascribed to the parent aromatic amine. Epidemiological studies (Gerarde and Gerarde, 1974; MacIntyre, 1975) were made on insufficient 3,3'-dichlorobenzidine operators to exclude this possibility.

Case et al. (1954) found 55 cases in all of 2-naphthylamine bladder cancer amongst the population of chemical workers, which they studied (see above), and there is other unequivocal evidence of 2-naphthylamine bladder cancer amongst rubber workers (Case and Hosker, 1954; Fox, Lindars and Owen, 1974). Bladder cancer was produced by this aromatic amine in dogs (Hueper, Wiley and Wolfe,

1938; Bonser, 1943), monkeys (Conzelman et al., 1969) and hamsters (Sellakumar, Montesano and Saffiotti, 1969). Hence, benzidine and 2-naphthylamine elicit bladder cancer in man and in certain species of animal.

In the early 1950s, M.H.C. Williams and colleagues became suspicious that 4-aminobiphenyl, which was also used in the dyestuff industry at that time, might be an additional source of human bladder cancer, and this supposition was confirmed by experiments in animals (Walpole, Williams and Roberts, 1952, 1954, 1955; Walpole and Williams, 1958). Out of a population of 315 American chemical workers who had been exposed to 4-aminobiphenyl, 53 of them eventually succumbed to bladder tumours (Melick et al., 1955; Melick, Naryka and Kelly, 1971).

Coal-tar, pitch and mineral-oil skin and lung cancer

Cancer of the skin, due to soot polycyclic aromatic hydrocarbons, was first described by Pott (1775), and since then coal tar (Volkmann, 1875), pitch (Manouviriez, 1876) and mineral oil (Bell, 1876) have been shown to be skin carcinogens. It might be mentioned here that coal tar was used as carcinogen in the first animal experiments. Yamagiwa and Ichikara (1915) painted it on to rabbits' ears for 11 years and, in later work, both Tsutsui (1918) and Murray (1921) produced similar results in mice by topical application.

Hammond et al. (1976) found that roofers, working with pitch, who had been occupationally exposed through the inhalation of benzo[α]pyrene (Cook, Hewett and Hieger, 1932), had a greatly enhanced susceptibility both to lung cancer and to cancer at several other sites, after a latent period of more than 20 years. This finding (Hammond et al., 1976) agrees with other ones (Lloyd, 1971; Doll, Vessey and Beasley, 1972), which showed that occupational exposure to benzo[α]pyrene was associated with increased mortality from lung cancer. Gas workers, exposed to products of coal carbonization, showed an increased incidence of lung cancer, 'topmen' on the retorts being particularly at risk (Doll et al., 1965).

The analysis of mineral lubricating-oil fractions was more troublesome than that of coal tar, largely because mineral oils contain a much more varied range of chemical substances than coal tar does, but benzo[α]pyrene was isolated (Tye, Graf and Horton, 1955) from cracked oil, and its presence was detected in the crude oil (Catchpole, MacMillen and Powell, 1971). The Medical Research Council (1968) reported on over 40 aromatic substances present in petroleum-oil fractions, but not many of them were found to be carcinogenic to animals when administered separately. Amongst metal workers in automatic machine shops, there was found to be an appreciable risk of skin cancer from oil in a survey undertaken in Birmingham, England (Cruikshank and Squire, 1950; Cruikshank and Gourevitch, 1952). Between 1950 and 1967, 187 cases of scrotal cancer occurred in the Birmingham area (Waterhouse, 1971). In 1966, for example, 16 out of 19 cases of scrotal cancer were caused by oil (Kipling, 1969). Metal rolling, tube drawing, metal hardening and general machine operating as well were proved to be sources of scrotal cancer from exposure to neat oils. Preventive measures have substantially reduced the incidence of skin cancers in industry (Kipling, 1974).

Asbestosis and bronchial carcinoma

Asbestosis, the fibrosis of the lung that is produced by inhalation of asbestos fibres, was detected in Britain and France at the turn of the century, but it was not until the late 1920s that asbestos was recognized as a major occupational hazard in the asbestos textile industry (Mereweather and Price, 1930). The first suspicion (1935) of an association between asbestos and bronchial carcinoma came from British and American pathologists, and this finding was reported in Britain first of all by the Ministry of Labour and National Service (1949). Fifteen per cent of all death certificates for males, which mentioned asbestosis, attributed death to bronchial carcinoma. Excessive risk was confirmed later by Doll (1955), who showed that those operators employed in scheduled occupations in asbestos textile factories before 1930, had a mortality rate for lung cancer which was 10 times higher than that of the background population. Later studies on this population showed that the incidence of carcinoma diminished with improved industrial hygiene. It followed that carcinoma of the lung was associated with severe pulmonary fibrosis, caused through heavy exposure to asbestos (Knox et al., 1968). Whilst asbestos dust had been shown (Wagner, Sleggs and Marchand, 1960) to cause diffuse mesotheliomas of the pleura and peritoneum, when (1964) mesotheliomas had been diagnosed in increasing number (Gilson, 1966), it was clear that, in general, asbestos workers had been exposed to more than one asbestos form. Thus, it was impossible to ascribe the exposure of any one operator to a particular form of asbestos.

Nickel respiratory cancer

Thirty years after the construction early this century of one of the world's largest nickel refineries (Mond process) at Clydach, Wales, 10 cases of nasal cancer were reported (Bridge, 1933) and, by 1948, 47 cases of nasal cancer and 82 cases of lung cancer had occurred there (Barrett, 1949). Doll examined death certificates in Britain for 1938–47 (Doll, 1958) and 1948–56 (Doll, 1957), and found that mortality for nasal cancer amongst nickel workers was 196 times that of the background population and that for lung cancer was 4.9 times higher. Workers employed in the Mond process suffered as much as 297 and 7.1 times the risk, respectively, of nasal and lung cancer than the general population. An older distribution for death from nickel cancer for 1948–56 compared with 1938–47 suggested that the greatest risk from nickel refining had occurred at some time in the past. (Amongst the operators who died in the 1948–56 period, there were no excess deaths from the two types of cancer in men under 50 years of age.) Morgan (1958) concluded that no excess deaths from lung or nasal cancer occurred amongst workers at Clydach who commenced their employment there after 1924, when the chemical plant was reconstructed and working conditions greatly improved.

Cigarette smoking and lung cancer

The presence of carcinogenic polycyclic aromatic hydrocarbons both in coal tar and in high boiling mineral-oil fractions suggested that the carcinogens might be present in tobacco smoke as well, especially as the aromatization of terpenoid constituents is known to occur at elevated temperatures. Three prospective studies on cigarette smoking in the 1950s (Doll and Bradford Hill, 1956; Hammond and Horn, 1958; Dorn, 1959) established beyond all reasonable doubt an association between smoking and lung cancer. Thus, in Hammond and Horn's work (1958), out of 190 000 white men between 50 and 69 years of age, nearly 12 000 had died by the end of 1955, 448 of them with primary cancer of the lung. Enhanced liability to lung cancer was clearly demonstrated amongst smokers, the risk increasing with increased exposure, i.e. with the numbers of cigarettes smoked. Doll, Bradford Hill and Kreyberg (1957) were able to show that lung cancer in non-smokers differed histologically from that occurring generally amongst heavy smokers. This fact supports the view that the two types of disease are due to different causes. Case (1958) pointed out that death rates from lung cancer were lower in summer than in winter, which reflects the prevalence of respiratory infection as a terminal event. It seems to have been established (Haenszel and Shimkin, 1956) that urban dwellers have a higher incidence of lung cancer than rural inhabitants, there being supposedly a linkage between the effects of heavy smoking and of atmospheric pollution in the towns. This contributive factor complicates the issue, and it seems probable that atmospheric pollution with soot and benzo[a]pyrene may even account for a proportion of the cases, otherwise attributable to smoking habits *per se*. Two observations support this supposition, viz. UK immigrants to New Zealand have a higher incidence of lung cancer than New Zealand-born persons of the same stock (Eastcott, 1956), and white male South Africans, who are amongst the heaviest smokers in the world, have a lower lung-cancer mortality rate than male British immigrants (Dean, 1959). Nevertheless, the association between heavy smoking and the induction of lung cancer seems to be unequivocal (Cornfield *et al.*, 1959).

Interestingly, prospective studies of the effects of smoking in human beings must rank amongst the most extensive experiments that have ever been made in animals or in man.

Benzene leukaemia

There is a growing suspicion that any substance, which damages bone-marrow function, may behave as a potential leukaemogen. The fact that benzene caused aplastic and hypoplastic anaemia has been known all of this century, and individual case histories have now revealed a correlation between exposure to benzene and the occurrence of leukaemia.

In the context of landmarks in our awareness of certain carcinogens, it is necessary to mention only some early observations. Thus, Delore and Borgomano (1928) diagnosed benzene leukaemia in an operator who had been so heavily (acutely) exposed to benzene that his contemporaries could not withstand more than two months' exposure without becoming ill. In 1932, Lignac (1932) produced 6 leukaemias and 2 infiltrating aleukaemic lymphoblastomas in 54 albino mice, which were given 0.001 ml of benzene in olive oil per week for 17–21 weeks: there were no cases of leukaemia in any of the 1500 control animals. Since then, there have been sporadic reports of acute and chronic leukaemia in human subjects which have been attributed to benzene poisoning. Thus, Penati and Vigliani (1938) and Vigliani (1938) collected together over the 1928–38 period 10 cases of benzene leukaemia, 60 cases of fatal aplastic anaemia and 4 other ones which did not appear to fit into either the anaemia or the leukaemia categories. In a series of papers (Bowditch and Elkins, 1939; Hunter, 1939; Mallory, Gall and Brickley, 1939), the occupational exposure to benzene involved 89 operators who were employed either in the manufacture of artificial leather or in making shoes with rubber welts containing benzene. Mallory, Gall and Brickley (1939) reported 19 cases (14 autopsies and 5 biopsies), including the 8 fatalities of Hunter (1939), which presented a blood picture, characterized by anaemia, leucopenia and thrombocytopenia. Two cases of leukaemia implicated a 28-year-old male (acute myeloblastic type) who had been exposed occupationally to benzene for 10 years, and a 12-year-old boy (lymphoblastic type) who had assisted in his father's paint shop 'for several years' removing paint from toys with a stripper known to contain benzene. By 1945, Saita had collected together another 23 cases of benzene leukaemia in which the acute forms predominated over chronic ones.

The most convincing cases of benzene leukaemia occurred in factories, concerned with the rotogravure process and shoe manufacturing, where there were outbreaks of chronic benzene poisoning. Many of these cases that occurred in Lombardy prior to 1963 were examined in Milano and Pavia (Vigliani and Saita, 1964). Out of 47 cases of benzene blood dyscrasias seen at Clinica de Lavoro, Milano, between 1942 and 1963, 6 were leukaemia, and of 41 cases of benzene blood dyscrasias examined at the Institute of Occupational Health in Pavia between 1961 and 1963, 5 were leukaemia. Thirteen additional cases of benzene leukaemia occurred in northern Italy between 1941 and 1963. Examination of insurance data for 1960–63 in Milano and Pavia revealed 11 cases of leukaemia amongst 68 blood dyscrasias, resulting from exposure to benzene.

Aflatoxin liver cancer

Dramatic loss of more than 100 000 turkey poults in Britain in 1960 led to the discovery that the fatal liver damage in these birds was due to carcinogenic secondary metabolites of *Aspergillus flavus* Link ex Fries, known as aflatoxins, which had contaminated the Brazilian groundnut meal that was fed to the turkeys (Lancaster, Jenkins and Philp, 1961; Sargeant *et al.*, 1961).

This finding is reminiscent of human disease attributable to mouldy yellowed rice (Uraguchi *et al.*, 1961), and the tragic effects of yellowed rice, imported into Japan after the Second World War (Enomoto and Saito, 1972; Uraguchi *et al.*, 1972).

The fact that aflatoxins are not only effective hepatotoxins, but were also found to be very potent hepatocarcinogens in experimental animals, led to their detailed investigation, the results of which have been reviewed (Kraybill and Shimkin, 1964; Wogan, 1965, 1966; Schoental, 1967; Goldblatt, 1969; Detroy, Lillehoj and Ciegler, 1971).

As the aflatoxins are the most potent hepatocarcinogens known, and as these mycotoxins contaminate such agricultural products as barley, cassava, cocoa, copra, cottonseed, groundnuts, maize, millet, oats, rice, sesame seeds, sorghum and tree nuts (pistachios etc.) particularly in the tropics, it became clear that the native population in those countries (Kenya, Mozambique, Swaziland, Thailand etc.) where these economic crops are harvested and stored, may present an incidence of dependent liver cancer. Field studies, which were made to assess a possible association with the occurrence of hepatomas in human subjects, established a significant correlation, and an intervention programme has been mounted to lower exposure and follow the downward trend of the disease (Linsell, 1979). While aflatoxins are partially correlated with the incidence of human hepatocellular cancer, the correlation is even better with hepatitis B. It seems that there is a synergism between viruses and chemicals.

The main problem raised by the awareness to widespread aflatoxin contamination is the protection of food supplies for the indigenous populations concerned.

Vinyl chloride angiosarcoma of the liver

A possible relationship between vinyl chloride exposure and human angiosarcoma of the liver first received attention in December 1973, when a case of this rare tumour was diagnosed at autopsy in a vinyl chloride worker from the B.F. Goodrich chemical plant at Louisville, Kentucky. This case was the third one that was recognized amongst vinyl chloride workers at this place, previous cases having been diagnosed in May 1970 and March 1973 (Creech and Johnson, 1974). The earliest recorded case (Heath, Falk and Creech, 1975) occurred in 1961; 5 other ones occurred in 1973/1974. In several instances, diagnosis of angiosarcoma of the liver was made after review of pathological material during the first part of 1974. All 13 of the cases that were considered in January 1975 by Heath, Falk and Creech (1975) had occurred amongst white male subjects; the time that elapsed between the start of work with vinyl chloride and diagnosis ranged from 12 to 29 years.

The reason why an aetiological association between vinyl chloride work and tumour induction could be inferred, initially on the basis of only 3 cases, is that the adventitious occurrence of angiosarcoma of the liver in human subjects is extremely rare. An expected annual incidence is of the order of 0.0014 cases/100000 or about 25–30 cases/year in the entire US population. Thus, about 0.03 cases of this tumour would be expected in the workforce concerned over a decade, and as 13 such cases had been recognized (Heath, Falk and Creech, 1975), a ratio of observed to expected cases of at least 400:1 was found.

At that time, 3 cases of vinyl chloride angiosarcoma of the liver had been identified in Germany (1969, 1971, 1974) (Marsteller *et al.*, 1973) and 2 cases in Sweden (Byrén and Holmberg, 1975).

These findings suggested that occupational exposure to vinyl chloride may cause hepatic fibrosis with angiosarcoma as a late manifestation, and this supposition was confirmed at a previous meeting in Lyon (IARC, 1974) at which 22 human cases of vinyl chloride angiosarcoma of the liver had been considered, including all 13 of the ones cited by Heath, Falk and Creech (1975) as well as one from Britain (1972) and one from Norway (1971), and also as a result of very extensive animal experiments, mostly with Sprague–Dawley rats and Swiss mice (Viola, Bigotti and Caputo, 1971; Maltoni and Lefemine, 1974a,b, 1975; Maltoni, 1976a,b,c, 1977a,b).

It is noteworthy that the human incidence of vinyl chloride angiosarcoma of the liver tended to plateau out after the initial reports (IARC, 1974; Heath, Falk and Creech, 1975), and never reached epidemic proportions. In retrospect, possibly only those operators who had formerly been responsible for the periodic descaling of the polymerization autoclaves were at risk. On-going epidemiological survey has witnessed decreased incidence of liver angiosarcoma amongst the vinyl chloride workforce, following the improved standards of hygiene which were introduced industry-wide as soon as the alarm had been raised (Creech and Johnson, 1974) of vinyl chloride being a human carcinogen.

Developing theory from its roots in experiment

Mutational theory

Following the discovery of the chromosomes and Boveri's (1914) suggestion that abnormal mitosis might be the cause of neoplasia, Bauer's (1928) mutational theory (Chapter 7) attributed new properties of the cancer cell, whilst maintaining its cellular variability, to a subtle change or changes in the cellular genome. This concept had much in its favour but, at that time, it could neither be proved nor disproved, as it was impossible to hybridize the putative mutated cell with a normal one and analyse the progeny. In addition, the possibility of seeking the correlation between mutagenesis and carcinogenesis which was inferred, was hampered by experiments in *Drosophila melanogaster* which was a difficult model to use for this purpose (Auerbach, 1939; Auerbach, Robson and Carr, 1947). Further progress awaited the development of genetically manipulated tester strains of bacteria (Ames *et al.*, 1973) (Chapters 2 and 7). Alongside developing theory, considerable progress was being made with the interaction between chemical carcinogens and cellular macromolecules *in vivo*.

The concept of metabolic activation

A considerable body of evidence suggested that carcinogens may require metabolic activation before they initiate carcinogenesis (Chapter 2). It might be argued that many carcinogens react with cellular nucleic acids and proteins in treated mammals and that, if chemical carcinogenesis involves such interaction, then metabolic activation would be essential, as many of them would not react *per se* with these macromolecules. Tissue specificity exposes the response of the highly differentiated mammalian body to chemical carcinogens and emphasizes the activation phenomenon (Chapter 2). Thus, for example, 2-naphthylamine, which causes bladder cancer in dogs and in man, proved to be entirely non-carcinogenic when implanted surgically in the bladder epithelium (Bonser and Jull, 1956), and it is non-carcinogenic to cats, rabbits and rats. Indirect evidence of metabolic activation comes from mutagenicity experiments (Ames *et al.*, 1953) in which many known carcinogens are active only where tests are made in the presence of drug-metabolizing enzymes. Other indirect evidence for the metabolic activation of chemical carcinogens derives from the inhibition of tumour induction by substances which either inhibit formation of reactive metabolites or induce their rapid disposition, or which provide alternative nucleophiles for preferential interaction with reactive metabolites (Chapter 5).

The search for reactive metabolites was hindered by the small proportion of them that was formed, in comparison with a larger proportion of detoxication products, such as the confusing array of phenols and their conjugates resulting from the metabolism of carcinogenic polycyclic aromatic hydrocarbons. On the other hand, modern chemical instrumentation, especially mass fragmentometry, greatly facilitates the present metabolite detection and identification. A milestone in the search for reactive carcinogen intermediates was the discovery of N-hydroxy compounds in the urine, containing the last of the carcinogen-related material, of rats given N-(2-fluorenyl)acetamide (Cramer, Miller and Miller, 1960) or 2-naphthylamine (Mason, 1976; Kadlubar, Miller and Miller, 1977). Intermediate epoxide formation would account for the metabolic products of polycyclic aromatic hydrocarbons (Boyland, 1950) and 25 years later, when reactive diol-epoxides had been found, molecular-orbital calculations were enlisted (Jerina and Lehr, 1977) to predict the most chemically reactive ones, obtainable from peri-condensed polycyclic aromatic hydrocarbons. Such diol-epoxides occur as *syn*- and *anti*-isomers and, for example in the case of benzo[a]pyrene, the (+)*anti*-7,8-dihydrodiol-9,10-epoxide is considered to be the most biologically potent (Slaga *et al.*, 1979). The discovery of epoxide metabolites has been important as well to monitoring the reactivity of vinyl chloride and the aflatoxins, but other reactive groups are important in this respect, and there might be cited the role of benzilic esters, as exemplified by a safrole metabolite.

The Millers' electrophilic theory

Much recent work on reactive carcinogen metabolites undoubtedly arose from the original proposal of the Millers (Miller, 1970; Miller and Miller, 1971), who attempted to account for the interaction of positively charged intermediates formed in N-(2-fluorenyl)acetamide and amino-azo dye metabolism, by the electrophilicity of ultimate reactive forms (that react at negatively charged nucleophilic centres in nucleic acids and proteins). Hathway (1980) showed that, in mammals, purely chemical reactions may occur in solution, if they are mechanistically favoured. Such chemical (non-enzymic) reactions, for example, account for the rearrangement of aliphatic carcinogen epoxides that are formed *in vivo*, and for interactions of reactive carcinogen intermediates with cellular macromolecules.

Interaction between reactive carcinogen intermediates and nucleic acid

Ten years later, in a discussion-type paper, Hathway and Kolar (1980) showed that the ensuing decade had vindicated the Millers' great unifying principle. These workers (Miller and Miller, 1971) attributed S_N1 mechanisms involving carbenium and nitrenium ions to reactions between N-(2-fluorenyl)acetamide or N-methylamino-azobenzene and DNA *in vivo*: the aromatic rings of the reagents permitted a distribution of charge, which conferred cation stability (Chapter 3). But, in general, there is no clear relation between reactivity of ultimate carcinogens and carcinogenic potency (Hathway and Kolar, 1980). Thus, initial reaction of vinyl chloride-related chloroethylene oxide or chloroacetaldehyde and the deoxyadenosine or deoxycytidine residues of DNA is S_N2, and the epoxy metabolite of aflatoxin B_1 reacts similarly with the deoxyguanosine residues, whereas the reactive form of safrole is a benzilic ester, which makes an S_N1 reaction with deoxyguanosine residues (Chapter 3).

Amongst direct-acting methylating carcinogens, dimethyl sulphate (DMS) and methyl methanesulphonate (MMS) show low electrophilic reactivity and are typical S_N2 alkylating agents, whereas N-methyl-N-nitrosurea (MNU), N-methyl-N'-nitro-N-nitrosoguanidine (MNNG) and 3-methyl-1-phenyltriazene (MPT) show coordination between the intermediate produced and the nucleophile, and a reactivity between that of an S_N1 and an S_N2 mechanism. Methylation by the latter agents probably involves Me-N_2^+ ions or methanediazohydroxide rather than the highly reactive Me$^+$ species (cited by Miller and Miller, 1971), and ought to be described as bimolecular. A mechanism is discussed in Chapter 2. The capacity of the agents to form O^6-methylguanine in target-tissue DNA correlates with their carcinogenic potency, and DES, DMS and MMS fail to induce tumours in tissues *in vivo* where MNU, N,N-dimethylnitrosamine (DMN), MPT and 3,3-dimethyl-1-phenyltriazene (DMPT) are active carcinogens. Indeed, the discovery of DMN as a strong carcinogen (1956) was a landmark in the recognition of chemical carcinogenesis. Again, nucleic acid is alkylated to a lesser extent by ethylating than by methylating agents. N,N-Diethylnitrosamine (DEN) and N-ethyl-N-nitrosurea (ENU) are much more powerful carcinogens than ethyl methane sulphonate (EMS). Strong biological evidence supports the chemical reaction of Cr^{VI} (or Cr^V)

with DNA *in vivo*. Like DES, DMS and MMS, *cis*-[PtCl$_2$(NH$_3$)$_2$] (II) reacts with DNA by an S$_N$2 mechanism.

Thus, very few reactions between ultimate chemical carcinogens and nucleic acid can be described as S$_N$1, and in the subject matter of this book, S$_N$2 reactions predominate over S$_N$1.

Qualitative application of Pearson's hardness–softness principle (Hathway and Kolar, 1980), which infers that the harder alkyl-N$_2^+$ cations would be expected to react with deoxyguanosine residues to give a larger proportion of O^6-alkylation products than the softer alkyl groups belonging to the DES, DMS and MMS agents, and that the softer (H$_3$N)$_2$Pt^{2+} cations would be expected to give almost exclusive N^7-platination, would have led to the same conclusions that the Millers (Miller and Miller, 1971) had reached.

Milestones in the 'oncogene' contribution

Of a number of cancer models, which had been proposed (Chapter 7), the one concerned with 'oncogenes' (Todaro and Huebner, 1972; Comings, 1973) appears to have been the most important. Two features might be mentioned, viz. the endogenous origin of the oncogenic (nucleotide) sequence and the discrete unit made by those DNA sequences which encode transformation and which appear to comprise an allelomorph of a normal cellular gene. This means that the transformation of normal cells into tumour cells would require the activation of specific cellular genes.

A model emerged which was used for the transformation of normal cellular genes into 'oncogenes' by viral regulation, and for this to apply to the similar transformation by chemical carcinogens, equivalent activation would have to be made through the rearrangement of blocks of normal cellular (nucleotide) sequences, following the modification of DNA by chemical carcinogens. In the chemical situation, the same genes would not necessarily be activated as the ones which were expropriated and activated by retroviruses.

Gene transfer was used (Shih *et al.*, 1979) (Chapter 7) as the tool for tackling the relevant problems, and the workers (Shih *et al.*, 1979) developed a technique from a method that had been used earlier by Graham and van der Eb (1973). The experimental evidence showed that the DNA, which had been modified by chemical carcinogen, was structurally different from the native DNA of the control cells. This difference must have to do with phenotype, as the oncogenic information conveyed by DNA transfer is bound to be responsible for the transformation phenotype in the donor cell-line (from which the DNA had been prepared). Modification of DNA occurs, therefore, in those regions of the cellular DNA genome which elicit a transformation phenotype.

Despite considerable progress (Chapter 7), it is uncertain how the possibility of what appears to be a single genetic change activating a mammalian transforming gene relates to the generally accepted multistage model (Chapter 6) for tumour induction. Strong evidence (Reddy *et al.*, 1982; Yuasa *et al.*, 1983) is forthcoming, however, that 'oncogene' activation is effected by a single point mutation of a DNA nucleotide residue for another one, which in turn resulted in misincorporation of a new amino acid residue instead of the normal one in the encoded protein, and that this conferred transforming properties on the gene product of the 'oncogene'. In recent work (Doolittle *et al.*, 1983; Waterfield *et al.*, 1983), a human endogenous protein, the platelet-derived growth factor (PDGT), which has known physiological effects on normal cells, has been identified as p^{28}sis, the putative transforming protein of the sis 'oncogene'. This finding emphasized the consistency of the genetic approach. The mitogenic cascades induced by such growth factors may link oncogenic function with the promotion of initiated cell types and a multistage process.

Concluding remarks

By exploring the biological significance of modified deoxynucleoside residues in the cellular DNA genome (Chapter 4), the inhibition of tumour induction (Chapter 5) and the mode of tumour promotion (Chapter 6), this book tentatively attempts to expose the common ground between the data presented by the modification of the cellular DNA genome by reactive carcinogen intermediates (Chapters 2 and 3) on the one hand and that by experimental genetics (Chapter 7) on the other.

Bibliography and references

AMES, B.N., DURSTON, W.E., YAMASAKI, E. and LEE, F.D. (1973) *Proc. Natl Acad. Sci. USA,* **70**, 2281
AUERBACH, C. (1939) *Proc. 7th Int. Congr. Genetics*, p. 51
AUERBACH, C., ROBSON, J.M. and CARR, J.G. (1947) *Science,* **105**, 243
BARRETT, G.P. (1949) *A Report of the Chief Inspector of Factories for 1948*. London: HMSO
BAUER, K.H. (1928) *Mutationstheorie der Geschwulst-Entstehung*. Berlin: Julius Springer
BELL, J. (1876) *Edinb. Med. J.,* **22**, 135
BILLIARD-DUCHESNE, J.L. (1959) *J. Urol. Med. Chir.,* **65**, 748
BONSER, G.M. (1943) *J. Pathol. Bacteriol.,* **55**, 1
BONSER, G.M. and JULL, J.W. (1956) *J. Pathol. Bacteriol.,* **72**, 489
BOVERI, T. (1914) *Zur Frage der Entstehung maligner Tumoren*. Jena: Gustav Fischer
BOWDITCH, M. and ELKINS, H.B. (1939) *J. Ind. Hyg. Toxicol.,* **21**, 321
BOYLAND, E. (1950) *Biochem. Soc. Symp.,* No. 5, 40
BRIDGE, J.C. (1933) *A Report of the Chief Inspector of Factories for 1932*. London: HMSO
BYRÉN, D. and HOLMBERG, B. (1975) *Ann. N.Y. Acad. Sci.,* **246**, 249
CASE, R.A.M. (1958) In *Carcinoma of the Lung*. Ed. J.R. Bignall. Chap. 11. Edinburgh: E & S Livingstone
CASE, R.A.M. and HOSKER, M.K. (1954) *Br. J. Prev. Med.,* **8**, 39
CASE, R.A.M., HOSKER, M.K., McDONALD, D.B. and PEARSON, J.T. (1954) *Br. J. Ind. Med.,* **11**, 75
CATCHPOLE, W.M., MACMILLEN, E. and POWELL, H. (1971) *Ann. Occup. Hyg.,* **14**, 171
COMINGS, D.E. (1973) *Proc. Natl Acad. Sci. U.S.A.,* **70**, 3324
CONZELMAN, G.M., MOULTON, J.E., FLANDERS, L.E., SPRINGER, K. and CROUT, D.W. (1969) *J. Natl Cancer Inst.,* **42**, 825
COOK, J.W., HEWETT, C. and HIEGER, I. (1932) *Nature,* **130**, 926
CORNFIELD, J., HAENSZEL, W., HAMMOND, E.C., LILIEMSELD, A.M., SHIMKIN, M.B. and WYNDER, E.L. (1959) *J. Natl Cancer Inst.,* **22**, 173
CRAMER, J.W., MILLER, J.A. and MILLER, E.C. (1960) *J. Biol. Chem.,* **235**, 885
CREECH, J.L. and JOHNSON, M.N. (1974) *J. Occup. Med.,* **16**, 150
CRUICKSHANK, C.N.D. and GOUREVITCH, A. (1952) *Br. J. Intern. Med.,* **9**, 74
CRUICKSHANK, C.N.D. and SQUIRE, J.R. (1950) *Br. J. Intern. Med.,* **7**, 1
DEAN, G. (1959) *Br. Med. J.,* **ii**, 852
DELORE, P. and BORGOMANO, C. (1928) *J. Med. Lyon,* **9**, 227
DETROY, R.W., LILLEHOJ, E.B. and CIEGLER, A. (1971) *Microbiol. Toxins,* **6**, 13
DOLL, R. (1955) *Br. J. Ind. Med.,* **12**, 81
DOLL, R. (1957) In *Industrial Pulmonary Diseases*. Eds E.J. King and C.M. Fletcher. p. 208. Boston: Little, Brown & Co.
DOLL, R. (1958) *Br. J. Ind. Med.,* **15**, 217
DOLL, R. and BRADFORD HILL, A. (1956) *Br. Med. J.,* **ii**, 1071
DOLL, R., BRADFORD HILL, A. and KREYBERG, L. (1957) *Br. J. Cancer,* **11**, 43

DOLL, R., FISHER, R.E.W., GAMMON, E.J., GUNN, W., HUGHES, G.O., TYRER, F.H. et al. (1965) *Br. J. Ind. Med.*, **22**, 1
DOLL, R., VESSEY, M.P. and BEASLEY, R.W.R. (1972) *Br. J. Ind. Med.*, **29**, 394
DOOLITTLE, R.F., HUNKAPILLER, M.W., HOOD, L.E., DEVARE, S.G., ROBBINS, K.C., AARONSON, S.A. et al. (1983) *Science*, **221**, 275
DORN, H.F. (1959) *Publ. Health Rep. (Wash.)*, **74**, 581
EASTCOTT, D.F. (1956) *Lancet*, **i**, 37
ENOMOTO, M. and SAITO, M. (1972) *Annu. Rev. Microbiol.*, **26**, 279
FOX, A.J., LINDARS, D.C. and OWEN, R. (1974) *Br. J. Ind. Med.*, **31**, 140
GERARDE, H.W. and GERARDE, D.F. (1974) *J. Occup. Med.*, **16**, 322
GILSON, J.C. (1966) *Trans. Soc. Occup. Med.*, **16**, 62
GOLDBLATT, L.A. (1969) *Aflatoxin, Scientific Background, Control and Implications.* New York: Academic Press
GOLDWATER, L.J., ROSSO, A.J. and KLEINFELD, M. (1965) *Arch. Environ. Health*, **11**, 814
GRAHAM, F.L. and VAN DER EB, A.J. (1973) *Virology*, **52**, 456
HAENSZEL, W. and SHIMKIN, M.B. (1956) *J. Natl Cancer Inst.*, **16**, 1417
HAMMOND, E.C. and HORN, D. (1958) *J. Am. Med. Assoc.*, **166**, 1294
HAMMOND, E.C., SELIKOFF, I.J., LAWTHER, P.L. and SEIDMAN, H. (1976) *Ann. N.Y. Acad. Sci.*, **271**, 116
HATHWAY, D.E. (1980) *Chem. Soc. Rev.*, **9**(1), 63
HATHWAY, D.E. and KOLAR, G.F. (1980) *Chem. Soc. Rev.*, **9**(2), 241
HEATH, C.W., FALK, H. and CREECH, J.L. (1975) *Ann. N.Y. Acad. Sci.*, **246**, 231
HUEPER, W.C., WILEY, F.H. and WOLFE, H.D. (1938) *J. Ind. Hyg. Toxicol.*, **20**, 46
HUNTER, F.T. (1939) *J. Ind. Hyg. Toxicol.*, **21**, 331
INTERNATIONAL AGENCY FOR RESEARCH ON CANCER (1974) *Internal Technical Report* No. 74/005, *Report of a Working Group on Vinyl chloride*. Lyon, France: IARC
JERINA, D.M. and LEHR, R.E. (1977) In *Microsomes and Drug Oxidations*. Eds V. Ulbrich, J. Roots, A. Hildebrandt, R.W. Estabrook and A.H. Conney. pp. 709–720. Proceedings of the Third International Symposium, Berlin, July 1976. Oxford: Pergamon
KADLUBAR, F.F., MILLER, J.A. and MILLER, E.C. (1977) *Cancer Res.*, **37**, 805
KIPLING, M.D. (1969) *Trans. Soc. Occup. Med.*, **19**, 39
KIPLING, M.D. (1974) *Ann. R. Coll. Surg.*, **55**, 79
KNOX, J.F., HOLMES, S., DOLL, R. and HILL, I.D. (1968) *Br. J. Ind. Med.*, **25**, 293
KRAYBILL, H.F. and SHIMKIN, M.B. (1964) *Adv. Cancer Res.*, **8**, 191
LANCASTER, M.C., JENKINS, F.P. and PHILP, J.M. (1961) *Nature*, **192**, 1095
LIGNAC, G.O.E. (1932) *Krankheitsforsch*, **9**, 426
LINSELL, C.A. (1979) In *Carcinogenic Risks: Strategies for Intervention*. Eds. W. Davis and C. Rosenfeld. International Agency for Research on Cancer Scientific Publications No. 25 (INSERM Symposia series Vol. 74). pp. 111–122. Lyon: IARC
LLOYD, J.W. (1971) *J. Occup. Med.*, **13**, 53
MACINTYRE, I. (1975) *J. Occup. Med.*, **17**, 23
MALLORY, T.B., GALL, E.A. and BRICKLEY, W.J. (1939) *J. Ind. Hyg. Toxicol.*, **21**, 355
MALTONI, C. (1976a) *Ann. N.Y. Acad. Sci.*, **271**, 431
MALTONI, C. (1976b) *Ann. N.Y. Acad. Sci.*, **271**, 444
MALTONI, C. (1976c) In *Environmental Pollution and Carcinogenic Risks*. Eds C. Rosenfeld and W. Davis. Institut National de la Santé et de la Recherche Médicale, Symposia Series, Vol. 52, pp. 127–149. International Agency for Research on Cancer, Scientific Publications, Vol. 13. Paris: Inserm
MALTONI, C. (1977a) In *Origins of Human Cancer*. Eds H.H. Hiatt, J.D. Watson and J.A. Winsten. Proc. Cold Spring Harbor Lab., Cold Spring Harbor, Massachusetts
MALTONI, C. (1977b) *Adv. Tumor Prev. Detect. Charact.*, **3**, 216
MALTONI, C. and LEFEMINE, G. (1974a) *Atti. Accad. naz. Lincei, Cl. Sci. Fis. Mat. Nat. Rend.*, [8] **56**, 1
MALTONI, C. and LEFEMINE, G. (1974b) *Environ. Res.*, **7**, 387
MALTONI, C. and LEFEMINE, G. (1975) *Ann. N.Y. Acad. Sci.*, **246**, 195
MANCUSO, T.F. and EL-ATTAR, A.A. (1967) *J. Occup. Med.*, **9**, 277
MANOUVIRIEZ, A. (1876) *Ann. Hyg. Publique*, **45**, 459
MANSON, D. (1976) In *Scientific Foundations of Oncology*. Eds T. Symington and R.L. Carter. pp. 281–291. London: Heinemann Medical
MARSTELLER, H.J., LELBACK, W.K., MÜLLER, R., JÜHE, S., LANGE, C.E., ROHNER, H.G. et al. (1973) *Dtsch. Med. Wochenschr.*, **98**, 2311
MEDICAL RESEARCH COUNCIL (1968) *Special Report Series*, **306**, 10. London: HMSO
MELEKA, F.M. (1983) *Dimensions of the Cancer Problem*. Basel: S. Karger
MELICK, W.F., ESCUE, H.M., NARYKA, J.J., MEZERA, R.A. and WHEELER, E.P. (1955) *J. Urol.*, **74**, 760

MELICK, W.F., NARYKA, J.J. and KELLY, R.E. (1971) *J. Urol.*, **106**, 220
MEREWEATHER, E.R.A. and PRICE, C.W. (1930) *Report on Effects of Asbestos Dust on the Lung, and Dust Suppression in the Asbestos Industry.* London: HMSO
MILLER, J.A. (1970) *Cancer Res.*, **30**, 559
MILLER, J.A. and MILLER, E.C. (1971) *J. Natl Cancer Inst.*, **47**, v
MINISTRY OF LABOUR AND NATIONAL SERVICE (1949) *A Report of the Chief Inspector of Factories for 1947 (CMD 7621).* London: HMSO
MORGAN, J.G. (1958) *Br. J. Ind. Med.*, **15**, 224
MURRAY, J.A. (1921) *Br. Med. J.*, **ii**, 795
PENATI, F. and VIGLIANI, E.C. (1938) *Rassegna Med. Indust.*, **9**, (5–6), 345
POTT, P. (1775) *Chirurgical Works.* Vol. 5, p.63. London: Hower, Clarke and Collins
REDDY, P.E., REYNOLDS, R.K., SANTOS, E. and BARBACID, M. (1982) *Nature*, **300**, 149
REHN, L. (1895) *Arch. Klin. Chir.*, **50**, 588
SAITA, G. (1945) *Med. Lavoro*, **36**, 143
SARGEANT, K., SHERIDAN, A., O'KELLY, J. and CARNAGHAN, R.B.A. (1961) *Nature*, **192**, 1096
SCHOENTAL, R. (1967) *Annu. Rev. Pharmacol.*, **7**, 343
SELLAKUMAR, A.R., MONTESANO, R. and SAFFIOTTI, U. (1969) *Proc. Am. Assoc. Cancer Res.*, **10**, 78
SHIH, C., SHILO, B., GOLDFARB, M.P., DANNENBERG, A. and WEINBERG, R.A. (1979) *Proc. Natl Acad. Sci. U.S.A.*, **76**, 5714
SLAGA, T.J., BRACKEN, W.J., GLEASON, G., LEVIN, W., YAGI, H., JERINA, D.M. et al. (1979) *Cancer Res.*, **39**, 67
SPITZ, S., MAGUIGAN, W.H. and DOBRINER, K. (1950) *Cancer*, **3**, 789
SÜSS, R., KINZEL, V. and SCRIBNER, J.D. (1970) *Krebs: Experimentellen und Konzepten.* pp. 1–3. Heidelberg: Springer-Verlag
TERRY REPORT (1964) *Cancer Mortality in the United States 1900–1960.* US Department of Health, Education and Welfare
TODARO, G.J. and HUEBNER, R.J. (1972) *Proc. Natl Acad. Sci. U.S.A.*, **69**, 1009
TSUTSUI, H. (1918) *Gann*, **12**, 17
TYE, R., GRAF, M.J. and HORTON, A.W. (1955) *Anal. Chem.*, **27**, 248
URAGUCHI, K., TATSUNO, T., SAKAI, F., TSUKIOKA, M., SAKAI, Y., YONEMITSU, O. et al. (1961) *Jap. J. Exp. Med.*, **31**, 19
URAGUCHI, K., SAITO, M., NOGUCHI, Y., TAKAHASKI, K., ENOMOTO, M. and TATSUNO, T. (1972) *Food Cosmet. Toxicol.*, **10**, 193
VIGLIANI, E.C. (1938) *Bericht, VIII Intern. Kongr. Unfallmed., Berufskrankh. Frankfurt.* p.825. Leipzig: Georg Thieme
VIGLIANI, E.C. and SAITA, G. (1964) *N. Engl. J. Med.*, **271**, 872
VIOLA, P.L., BIGOTTI, A. and CAPUTO, A. (1971) *Cancer Res.*, **31**, 516
VOLKMANN, R. (1875) *Beitr. Chirurg. Leipzig*, 370
WAGNER, J.C., SLEGGS, C.A. and MARCHAND, P. (1960) *Br. J. Ind. Med.*, **17**, 260
WALPOLE, A.L. and WILLIAMS, M.H.C. (1958) *Br. Med. Bull.*, **14**, 141
WALPOLE, A.L., WILLIAMS, M.H.C. and ROBERTS, D.C. (1952) *Br. J. Ind. Med.*, **9**, 255
WALPOLE, A.L., WILLIAMS, M.H.C. and ROBERTS, D.C. (1954) *Br. J. Ind. Med.*, **11**, 105
WALPOLE, A.L., WILLIAMS, M.H.C. and ROBERTS, D.C. (1955) *Br. J. Cancer*, **9**, 170
WATERFIELD, M.D., SCRANCE, G.T., WHITTLE, N., STROOBANT, P., JOHNSSON, A., WASTESON, A. et al. (1983) *Nature*, **304**, 35
WATERHOUSE, J.A.H. (1971) *Ann. Occup. Hyg.*, **14**, 161
WOGAN, G.N. (ED.) (1965) *Mycotoxins in Foodstuffs.* Cambridge, USA: MIT
WOGAN, G.N. (1966) *Bacteriol. Rev.*, **30**, 460
YAMAGIWA, K. and ICHIKAWA, K. (1915) *J. Jap. Pathol. Ges.*, **5**, 142
YUASA, Y., SRIVASTAVA, S.K., DUNN, C.Y., RHIM, J.S., REDDY, P.E. and AARONSON, S.A. (1983) *Nature*, **303**, 775

Chapter 2

Activation of chemical carcinogens in the mammal

On purely chemical grounds, the likelihood that many notable chemical carcinogens react *per se* with cellular nucleic acids and proteins is slight. Yet, a considerable body of evidence indicates that such reactions occur in treated animals (*see* Chapter 3) and that the resulting miscoding events during DNA synthesis predispose the tissue in question towards malignancy (*see* Chapter 4). These two statements are incongruent, but both appear to be true, and both must be taken into account. The paradox is more readily understandable if chemical carcinogens are transformed *in vivo* into more highly reactive intermediates prior to reaction with target-organ nucleic acid and the induction of tumours. This chapter presents the evidence for this assumption and explores whether the formation of reactive (carcinogen) metabolites *de novo* mirrors tissue specificity.

Presumptive evidence of metabolic activation

Tissue specificity

Tissue specificity, more than anything else, reflects the response of the mammalian body towards chemical carcinogens, and it ought to be considered that the majority of actual chemical substances, which are known to be carcinogenic to man, were discovered through intensive investigations following the specific diagnosis of occupational cancer. Whilst sometimes tissue specificity has wide interspecies significance and, for example, vinyl chloride causes liver cancer in all of the mammalian species, including man, which have ever been exposed, regardless of the route of entry (Viola, Bigotti and Caputo, 1971; Maltoni and Lefemine, 1974a,b, 1975; Maltoni, 1976a,b,c, 1977a,b), in other cases, tissue specificity is combined with species specificity and, for example, β-naphthylamine promotes bladder cancer in dogs, hamsters and monkeys and in man, but produces hepatomas in mice, and is non-carcinogenic to cats, rabbits and rats (Clayson, 1975; Shubik and Clayson, 1976). In general, after enteral administration of a dose of a foreign compound, the greatest concentration of unchanged substance will be present in the mouth and stomach, and this applies to operatives exposed occupationally to β-naphthylamine. Tumours were induced in this case, however, at sites remote from those biological situations. They developed either at the principal sites of metabolism, and foreign compound metabolizing capacity occurs in the following descending order liver > kidneys > lungs, or in those organs, like the bladder, that are concerned with the excretion of foreign compound-related material. Thus, it would appear that some form of metabolic activation is essential for β-naphthylamine to express its carcinogenic potential. The lack of carcinogenicity, which has been demonstrated in three mammalian species (*see above*), supports the idea of metabolic activation occurring in those mammals where β-naphthylamine is a frank carcinogen.

Whilst lipid-soluble polycyclic aromatic hydrocarbons, such as benzo[α]pyrene, which occurs in soot, cause skin cancer (Pott, 1775; Yamagiwa and Ichikawa, 1915; Tsutsui, 1918; Bloch and Dreifuss, 1921; Cook, Hewett and Hieger, 1933), and metal carcinogens like nickel (Chief Inspector of Factories, 1933, 1952; Doll, 1958; Morgan, 1958; Williams, 1958; Sunderman, 1968; Doll, Morgan and Speizer, 1970) and chromium (Gross and Kolsch, 1943; Letterer, Neidhardt and Klett, 1944; Machle and Gregorius, 1948; Baetjer, 1950; Mancuso and Hueper, 1951; Brinton, Frasier and Koven, 1952; Spannagel, 1953; Bidstrup and Case, 1956; Goodgame, Hayman and Hathway, 1982) provoke lung (nose) cancer, there is a strong supposition that these carcinogens are metabolized by the skin and lung tissues respectively via the percutaneous and inhalational routes. Clearly, vinyl chloride (*see above*), N,N-dimethylaminophenylazobenzene (Butter Yellow) (Kensler, Dexter and Rhoads, 1942; Druckrey and Küpfmüller, 1949; Druckrey, 1959; Williams, 1962) and N,N-dimethylnitrosamine (Druckrey and Schmähl, 1962; Druckrey *et al.*, 1963; Le Page and Christie, 1969), which are potent hepatocarcinogens, act at the major site of metabolism. Similar reasoning holds also for other important carcinogens, such as the aromatic amines, 4-aminobiphenyl, benzidine and 2-fluorenylacetamide (2AAF), the amino-azo dyes, the plant products cycasin and safrole (*see below*) and the microbiological products including the aflatoxins.

Despite its limitations, the foregoing evidence gave rise to the idea that chemical carcinogens, in general, are converted into highly reactive molecular forms *in vivo*.

Physiological systems for testing localized carcinogenic activity

The possibility of using physiological preparations to assist the localized testing of procarcinogenic metabolites is shown clearly in connection with the investigation of β-naphthylamine bladder cancer. At first sight, the evidence suggests that the induction of bladder cancer is complex, as the bladder is not a major site of foreign compound metabolism, and as treated mice and rats do not develop bladder cancer. It was found at an early stage in the work (Hueper, Wiley and Wolfe, 1938; Bonser, 1943; Bonser *et al.*, 1956), however, that systematically treated dogs provided an effective experimental model, and the possibility that a reactive β-naphthylamine metabolite might be transported to the bladder (*see* Miller, 1970) suggested a way of tackling this problem (Clayson, 1962). Accordingly, in this subsection, the use of physiological systems and the resulting evidence is discussed in the context of β-naphthylamine bladder cancer.

A paraffin or cholesterol pellet containing the test substance was surgically implanted in the bladder lumen of mice (Bonser and Jull, 1956; Clayson and Pringle, 1961; Clayson and Cooper, 1970; Clayson, 1974). Initial experiments were disappointing, however, the case of 2-amino-1-naphthylsulphate being equivocal, but at any rate β-naphthylamine *per se* and some other hydroxy-2-naphthylamine derivatives proved to be entirely non-carcinogenic. *N*-(2-Naphthyl)hydroxylamine was shown eventually by surgical implantation in the bladders of mice (*see above*) to be important to β-naphthylamine bladder cancer (Bonser *et al.*, 1963; Bryan, Brown and Price, 1964). Both *N*-(2-naphthyl)hydroxylamine and another β-naphthylamine metabolite, 2-nitrosonaphthalene, proved to be carcinogenic in dogs (Deichmann and Radomski, 1969). Finally, a good correlation was established between the induction of tumours in dogs and the presence of N-oxidation products of the parent aromatic amine in the urine (Radomski and Brill, 1971).

The fact that repeated installation of *N*-(2-naphthyl)hydroxylamine into the bladders of dogs produced tumours (Radomski and Brill, 1970) indicates strongly (but does not prove) that, in animals treated systematically with β-naphthylamine, *N*-(2-naphthyl)hydroxylamine would have initiated bladder cancer by invasion from the lumen rather than from the serosal side of the epithelial cells. An alternative experiment in which dogs with a catheterized ureter are treated systematically with a protected form of *N*-(2-naphthyl)hydroxylamine does not appear to have been made.

Mutagenicity testing

The indirect evidence that many chemical carcinogens gave a positive response in the Ames test (*see below*) only in the presence of metabolizing enzymes (*Table 2.1*) is relevant to the present discussion on the metabolic activation of chemical carcinogens *de novo*. During the 1970s, sensitive bacterial strains began to be employed to diagnose mutagens and, as a result of outstanding progress in genetics, Ames and his colleagues (Ames, 1971, 1972; Ames, Sims and Grover, 1972; Ames *et al.*, 1972, 1973; Ames, Lee and Durston, 1973; Durston and Ames, 1974; Kier, Yamasaki and Ames, 1974; Ames, Kammer and Yamasaki, 1975; Ames, McCann and Yamasaki, 1975; McCann *et al.*, 1975b; McCann and Ames, 1976) developed a system which utilized a special set of histidine-deficient mutants of *Salmonella typhimurium* together with mammalian microsomal enzymes. By means of this test, nearly all of several hundred carcinogenic substances examined proved to be mutagens, and almost no non-carcinogens were mutagenic. It follows from these studies that most chemical carcinogens seem to cause cancer through somatic mutation. Both in the case of bacterial mutagenicity (q.v.) and in that of mammalian cancer, active carcinogen metabolites react with somatic DNA.

TABLE 2.1. Mutagenicity tests

Carcinogen	Salmonella typhimurium *tester* strain plus metabolic activation	References	Unique type of DNA damage
Vinyl chloride	TA100, TA1530 or TA1535	McCann *et al.* (1975b) Malaveille *et al.* (1975) Rannug, Göthe and Wachtmeister (1976) Rannug *et al.* (1974)	Base-pair substitution
Aromatic amines	TA98, TA1537 or TA1538	Ames *et al.* (1973)	Frame-shift
Dialkylnitrosamines	TA1530	Bartsch, Malaveille and Montesano (1976)	Base-pair substitution
Cr^{VI}	TA100 or TA1535 and TA98 or TA1537		Base-pair substitution and frame-shift
Cr^{3+}			None

Inhibition of tumour initiation

Indirect evidence for the metabolic activation of chemical carcinogens stems also from the inhibition or prevention of neoplasia (Wattenberg, 1978). Thus, granted the key importance of foreign compound metabolism to tumour induction, the administration of specific substances before or simultaneously with the carcinogen might be expected theoretically to (a) inhibit the pathway leading to metabolic activation, (b) scavenge free radical intermediates, (c) accelerate the pathway of active metabolite disposal, and/or (d) compete selectively with DNA as substrate for reactive carcinogen metabolites by supplying alternative nucleophiles (Hathway, 1979). Whilst empirical discovery of the inhibition of tumour initiation (Wattenberg, 1978) outstrips its rationalization in molecular terms, a considerable body of evidence (Goodgame, Trosko and Yager, 1976; Lam and Wattenberg, 1977; Slaga and Bracken, 1977; Weisburger, Evarts and Wenk, 1977) infers that the inhibitory effect of BHT (3,5-di-*tert*-butyl-4-hydroxytoluene) and other antioxidants in this respect is exerted before any damage to DNA takes place (*see* Chapter 5).

Reactive metabolites of chemical carcinogens

Aromatic amines

Nitrogen hydroxylation, to which reference has been made in the preceding section of this chapter, has been shown to be a prerequisite for the induction of bladder cancer by this series of compounds. The resulting *N*-arylhydroxylamine might be further esterified in some, but probably not all, cases. The ultimate carcinogen is unstable and affords a highly reactive electrophile (*Scheme 2.1*), which reacts with somatic DNA (*see* Chapter 3). It might be mentioned here that, in these compounds, the aromatic rings concerned permit a distribution of charge which confers cation stability (*Scheme 2.2*). Whilst the N-hydroxy derivatives of primary aromatic amines, such as α- and β-naphthylamines and 4-aminobiphenyl, are unstable and are readily oxidized to the corresponding arenenitroso compounds, the N-hydroxy derivatives of acylated aromatic amines, such as 2AAF, are relatively more stable. Hence, the latter N-hydroxy derivatives are more amenable to detection and isolation. It is relevant that the first metabolically formed

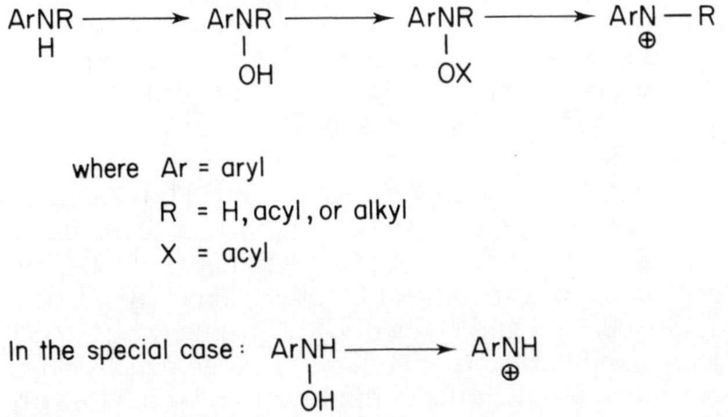

$$\text{ArNRH} \longrightarrow \text{ArNR} \mid \text{OH} \longrightarrow \text{ArNR} \mid \text{OX} \longrightarrow \text{ArN}^{\oplus}\text{—R}$$

where Ar = aryl
R = H, acyl, or alkyl
X = acyl

In the special case: $\text{ArNH} \mid \text{OH} \longrightarrow \text{ArNH}^{\oplus}$

Scheme 2.1

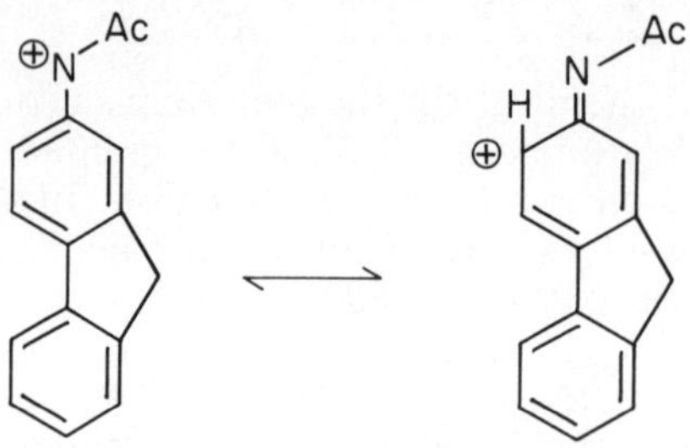

Scheme 2.2

arylhydroxylamine to be identified was N-hydroxy-N-(2-fluorenyl)acetamide (Cramer, Miller and Miller, 1960) in the glucuronidase-treated late urines of rats dosed with 2AAF.

In connection with these findings, it is salutary to remember that: (a) Leuenberger (1912) first proposed over 70 years ago that hydroxylamines may be the causative (carcinogen) metabolites of aniline bladder cancer; (b) in relation to methaemoglobinaemia, Heubner (1913) suggested the biological N-hydroxylation of aromatic amines; (c) 2-amino-1-naphthol was identified over 60 years ago in the urine of dogs treated with β-naphthylamine (Engel, 1920). Moreover, early this century, N-(2-naphthyl)hydroxylamine and N-(4-biphenyl)hydroxylamine had been prepared chemically from the parent amines by the Willstätter school in Zürich (Willstätter and Kubli, 1908).

A clue to the possible occurrence of an esterification step in the metabolic activation of aromatic amines (*Scheme 2.1*) was provided by Poirier et al. (1967) who, failing to prepare the unstable N-hydroxy derivative (1) (*Scheme 2.3*) N-4-methylamino-azobenzene (MAB), synthesized instead the benzoyloxy ester (2). Reaction of (2) with various amino acids and peptides *in vitro* gave covalently bound products (*Scheme 2.3*), similar to the ones obtained through the hydrolysis of the liver proteins of rats which had been dosed with MAB.

Although various synthetic esters of N-hydroxy-2AAF were prepared and were shown to be reactive, they would not appear to be generated in the cell *in vivo*. This stimulated the investigation of N-sulphates (De Baun et al., 1968; King and Phillips, 1968; De Baun, Miller and Miller, 1970), formed from N-hydroxy-2AAF by 3'-phosphoadenosine-5'-phosphosulphate (PAPS) in the presence of an enzyme in the hepatocyte cytosol. The tumorogenicity of the resulting N-sulphate was not really what would have been expected, however, and this may have been due to ester breakdown by its reaction with cellular nucleophiles before the N-sulphate reached critical cell sites. In this connection, it was found that acetanilide reduces the carcinogenicity of 2AAF by depletion of intracellular SO_4^{2-} concentration (Yamamoto et al., 1968; Weisburger et al., 1972), and that simultaneous administration of SO_4^{2-} with N-hydroxy-2AAF increases the reactivity and toxicity of the latter metabolite (De Baun et al., 1968).

The nature of the ester or esters of N-hydroxy-2AAF, which is (are) produced *de novo* is not, however, clearcut, and whilst a great deal of biochemical data has been generated on the metabolism and metabolic activation of 2AAF, much of which is more or less pertinent to its mechanism of carcinogenicity, the papers by Dybing and Soederlund (1978), Dybing, Soederlund and Haug (1979), Dybing et al. (1979) and Stout and Backer (1979) are landmarks. In familiar cell systems, Dybing, Soederlund and Haug (1979) demonstrated the effect of inducers and inhibitors on

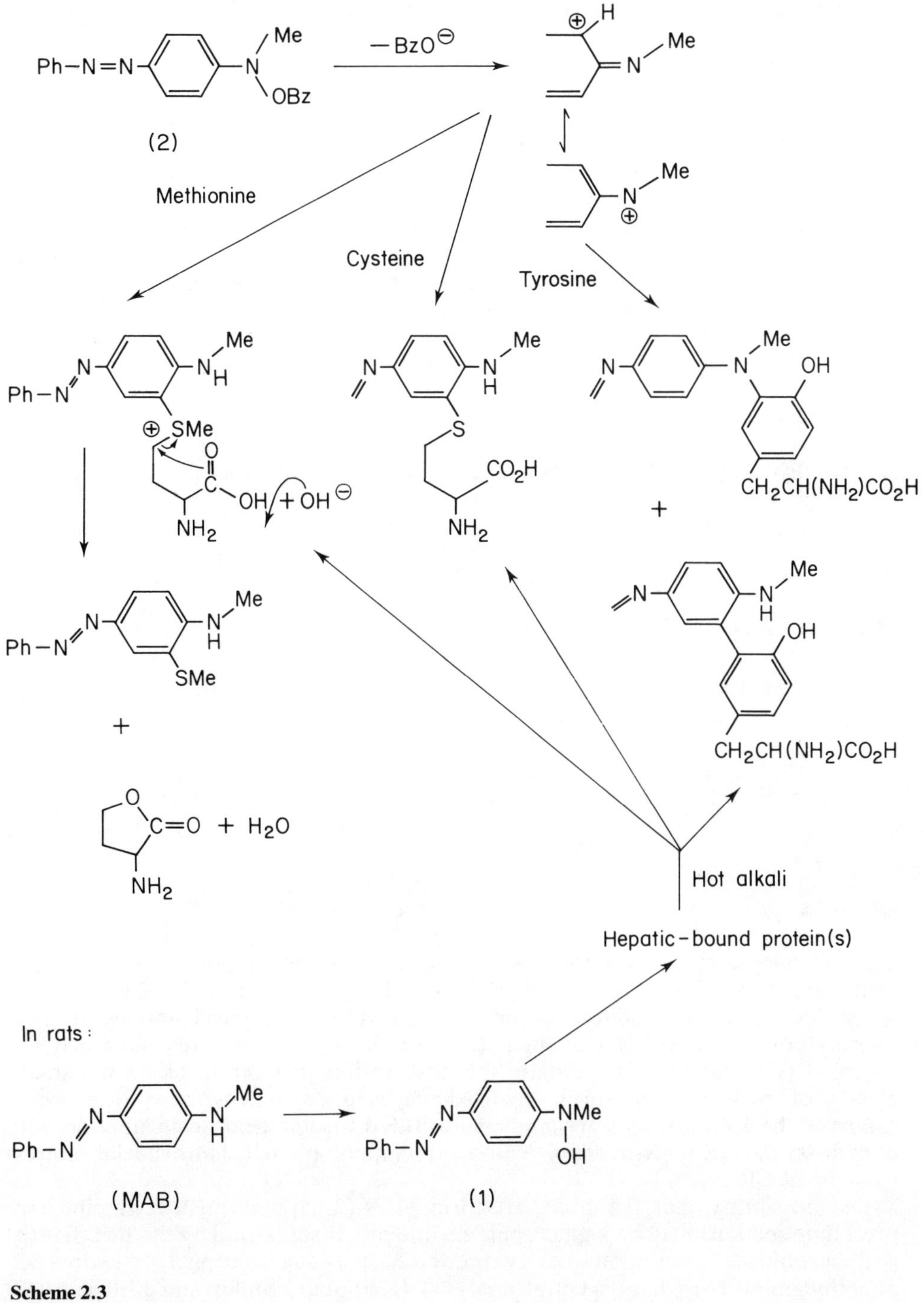
Ph–N=N–
Me
N
OBz
– BzO⊖
(2)
Methionine
Cysteine
Tyrosine
Me
N
Me
N
⊕
SMe
O
C
OH
+ OH ⊖
NH₂
S
CO₂H
NH₂
OH
CH₂CH(NH₂)CO₂H
+
SMe
+
C=O + H₂O
NH₂
Hot alkali
Hepatic-bound protein(s)
In rats:
NMe
OH
(MAB)
(1)

Scheme 2.3

the oxidation, deacetylation and conjugation of 2AAF. Formation of the relatively unimportant alicyclic hydroxylated 9-hydroxy-2AAF was neither induced by pre-treatment with β-naphthoflavone nor inhibited by that with *p*-nitrophenol. Addition of microsomes increased the mutagenicity of 2AAF, possibly through deacetylation of *N*-hydroxy-2AAF to *N*-hydroxy-2-aminofluorene, but not of 2-aminofluorene (*see also* Dybing and Soederlund, 1978; Stout and Becker, 1979). Using separate human-liver subcellular components, Dybing *et al.* (1979) found that both the *in vitro* mutagenicity of 2AAF and the degree of N-hydroxylation corresponded with those of 2-aminofluorene. Human liver microsomal and cytosol fractions metabolized *N*-hydroxy-2AAF into mutagens, presumably through deacetylation. Dybing *et al.* (1979) referred to a poor correlation between the extent of the covalent binding of 2AAF with liver microsomal protein and the degree of mutagenicity in the Ames test. But, there is no reason at all (present author) why binding of reactive 2AAF metabolites with liver microsomal proteins should be connected with the determinative transformation of bacterial DNA (by not necessarily the same 2AAF metabolites) that led to the reversion found in the mutagenicity testing.

It is of very great interest that Lhoest, Roberfroid and Mercier (1978) have investigated the ring–chain tautomerism (Baker, 1934) of *N*-acetyl-2-fluorenylhydroxylamine (3) (*Scheme 2.4*) involving the structures (3)–(5). This

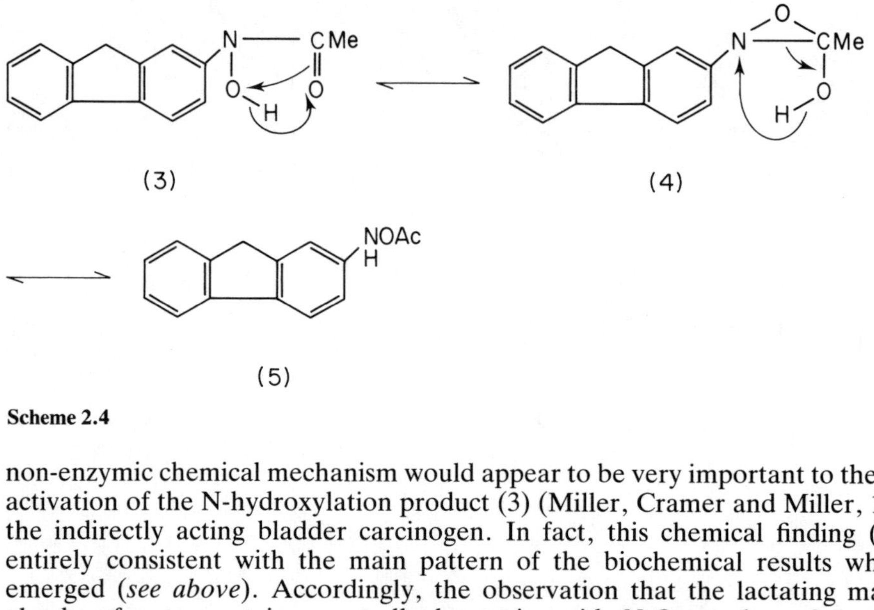

Scheme 2.4

non-enzymic chemical mechanism would appear to be very important to the further activation of the N-hydroxylation product (3) (Miller, Cramer and Miller, 1960) of the indirectly acting bladder carcinogen. In fact, this chemical finding (q.v.) is entirely consistent with the main pattern of the biochemical results which has emerged (*see above*). Accordingly, the observation that the lactating mammary glands of rats contain an arylhydroxamic acid *N,O*-acetyltransferase which catalyses the formation of arylamine-substituted nucleic acid on incubation with *N*-hydroxy-2AAF or *N*-hydroxy-*N*-(4-acetyl)aminobiphenyl, is of special interest (King *et al.*, 1979).

The possibility that the transport form of *N*-(2-naphthyl)hydroxylamine (*see* preceding section) may be a glucuronide conjugate is supported by the fact that (*a*) β-glucuronidase treatment of synthetic *N*-(β-1-glucosiduronyl)-*N*-hydroxy-2-naphthylamine (6) (mass spectral analysis) (Kadlubar, Miller and Miller, 1977)

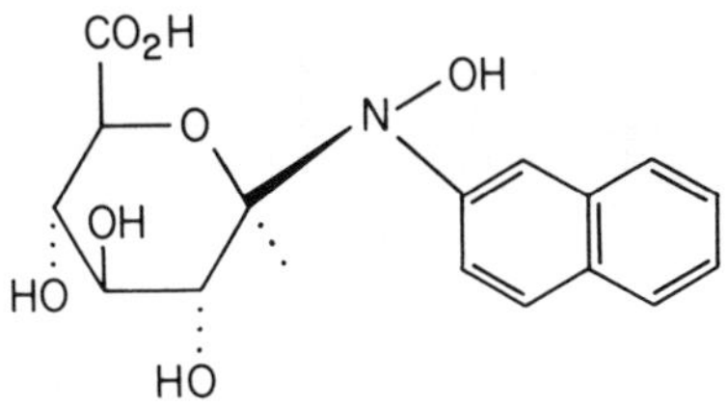

(6)

regenerated *N*-(2-naphthyl)hydroxylamine quantitatively and (*b*) that *N*-(2-naphthyl)hydroxylamine decomposed under acidic conditions to give arylnitrenium ions which reacted with nucleic acids (Kadlubar, Miller and Miller, 1977). Hence, hepatically synthesized (6) is now considered to be the transport form of β-naphthylamine, which delivers *N*-(2-naphthyl)hydroxylamine to the bladder, where electrophiles are produced in the normally acidic urine of dogs and of man. Kadlubar, Miller and Miller (1977) found that *N*-hydroxy-1-naphthylamine, *N*-hydroxy-2-naphthylamine and *N*-hydroxy-4-aminobiphenyl and their glucuronides were relatively stable and unreactive at neutral pH, but at pH 5, (6) and the presumed glucuronides of *N*-hydroxy-1-naphthylamine and *N*-hydroxy-4-aminobiphenyl were hydrolysed rapidly to the corresponding *N*-arylhydroxylamines, which were converted into reactive intermediates (*see above*). The glucuronide conjugate of *N*-hydroxy-4-aminobiphenyl has been isolated in a pure form from the urine of treated dogs by molecular size, ion-exchange, adsorption and partition chromatography (Radomski *et al.*, 1977). The dog metabolite was equivalent in all respects to *N*-(4-biphenyl)-*N*-hydroxy-D-glucuronosylamine (7) (Radomski *et al.*, 1977), synthesized direct from *N*-hydroxy-4-aminobiphenyl and glucuronic acid (Boyland, Manson and Orr, 1957), and differed from (*N*-(4-biphenyl)hydroxylamine-β-D-glucopyranoside)uronate (8), synthesized (Conrow and Bernstein, 1971) by Königs–Knorr synthesis (1900). Radomski *et al.* (1977) concluded that, since (7) and the parent *N*-hydroxy-4-aminobiphenyl are active mutagens in *S. typhimurium* strains TA1538 and TA98, but not in TA1535 and TA1537, (7) is the transport form of 4-aminobiphenyl, which delivers *N*-hydroxy-4-aminobiphenyl to the bladder.

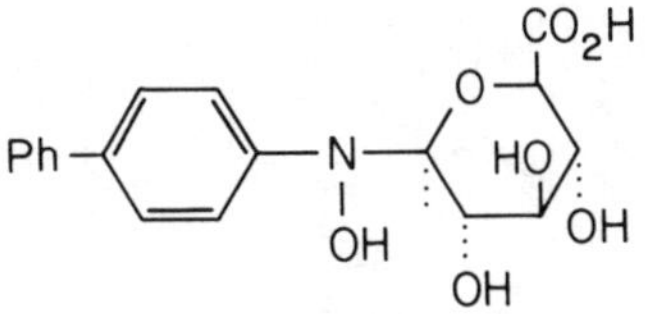

(7) 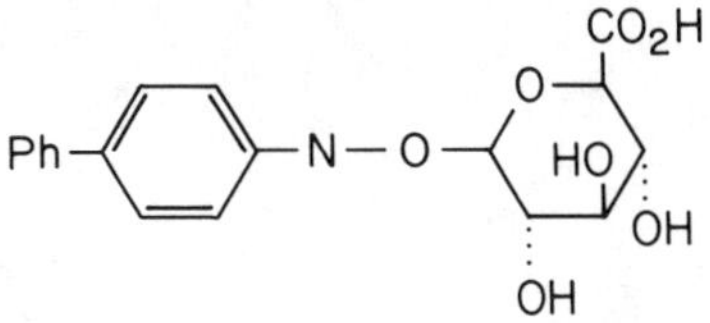 (8)

Amino-azo dyes

Some members of the huge array of azo dyes are undoubtedly mutagens and potent carcinogens, but others appear to be innocuous, and Hathway (1984a) in an attempt to rationalize this problem suggested three categories. In the first, where the reaction product of azo reductase contains a carcinogenic aromatic amine, the formation of this compound *de novo* appears to account for the carcinogenicity of

(9)

(10)

(11)

(12)

(13)

the original dyestuffs. Thus, for example, Ponceau 3R (9) affords 2,4,5-trimethylaniline, which is a mutagen in the Ames test (Hartman, Andrews and Chung, 1979), and which caused hepatomas and lung adenomas in CD mice (Feller, Morita and Gillette, 1971). Compound (9) is a hepatocarcinogen in rats (Grice, Mannell and Allmark, 1961; Hansen et al., 1963; Mannell, 1964) and causes bladder tumours in mice (Bonser et al., 1963). Similarly, trypan blue (10) affords o-tolidine (3,3'-dimethylbenzidine), which is a mutagen in the Ames test (Hartman, Fulk and Andrews, 1978), and which is a systemic carcinogen in rats (Pliss, 1965; Pliss and Zabezhinsky, 1970). In rats, (10) produces reticulum-cell sarcomas, particularly of the liver, as well as fibrosarcomas at the site of injection (Simpson, 1952; Marshall, 1953; Oka et al., 1957; Ooneda et al., 1957; Brown and Norlind, 1959, 1961; Ito and Farber, 1966; Papacharalampous, 1966). Direct Black 38 (11), Direct Blue 6 (12) and Direct Brown 95 (13) all give the human bladder carcinogen, benzidine and its N-acetyl and N,N'-diacetyl derivatives as metabolites *in vivo* (Scott, 1952; Case et al., 1954; von Übelin and Pletscher, 1954; Goldwater, Rosso and Kleinfeld, 1965; Mancuso and El-Attar, 1967). All three amino-azo dyes are powerful hepatocarcinogens in rats (IARC, 1982). Furthermore, Direct Black 38 was a mutagen in *S. typhimurium* strains TA98 and TA100 when tested in the presence of mouse-liver microsomes (Lazear et al., 1979), and urine from treated rats was also mutagenic in these *S. typhimurium* strains (Nony et al., 1980; Tanaka, 1980). An epidemiological study of silk dyers and painters, who had suffered multiple exposure both to benzidine-based dyes and to others, showed that these exposures were strongly associated with the incidence of bladder cancer observed (IARC, 1982).

In the second class, where azo reductase does not afford carcinogenic aromatic amines, and where the azo dyes themselves are carcinogens, the carcinogenicity of the parent compounds seems to derive from direct N-hydroxylation of the dyes *per se*. The lipophilicity of this group of compounds and the consequent tissue retention contribute to the hydroxylation mechanism. Reference has been made in the preceding subsection of this chapter to the case of p-methylamino-azobenzene (MAB) (*Scheme 2.3*), and further exemplification is provided by the hepatocarcinogens, p-amino-azobenzene (14) (Kirby, 1947; Kirby and Peacock, 1947; Odashima and Hashimoto, 1968), p-dimethylamino-azobenzene (DAB) (15) (Druckrey, 1943, 1951; Druckrey and Küpfmüller, 1948), o-amino-azotoluene (16) (Yoshida, 1932, 1933; Sasaki and Yoshida, 1935), chrysoidine (17) (Albert, 1956) and para-Red (18). *p*-Dimethylamino-azobenzene (15) and *o*-amino-azotoluene (16) caused bladder cancer in dogs (Nelson and Woodward, 1953). After β-glucuronidase treatment, the urine of rats dosed (15) was mutagenic to *S. typhimurium* TA1538 (Commoner, Vithayathil and Henry, 1974), and (14) was shown to be a mutagen in the same bacterial strain (Ames, 1973).

In the third category, where there is a relatively high degree of sulphonation in comparison with molecular size as, for example, in the case of Amaranth (19), Sunset Yellow FCF (20), Orange G (21) and Ponceau SX (22), detergent activity opposes absorption from the gut and facilitates the rapid elimination from the body of any unchanged dye which has been absorbed. Thus, little, if any, risk is incurred from the use of these compounds (*see* IARC, 1975). The parallel between this group of innocuous azo dyes and the non-carcinogenic β-naphthylamine sulphonic acid derivatives, such as Tobias acid, 2-naphthylamine-1-sulphonic acid, and Brönner acid, 2-naphthylamine-6-sulphonic acid, is noteworthy.

Nitrosamines

Direct-acting methylating agents, such as *N*-methyl-*N*-nitrosourea (MNU), *N*-methyl-*N'*-nitro-*N*-nitrosoguanidine (MNNG) and 3-methyl-1-phenyltriazene (MPT), contain the R–N–N–O or R–N–N–N system, and they show a coordination between the intermediate produced and the nucleophile, which lies between that of Ingold's S_N1 and S_N2 categories (Garrett and Goto, 1973) with a Swain–Scott s-value of 0.42 (Veleminsky, Osterman-Golkar and Ehrenberg, 1970; Osterman-Golkar, 1974). Hathway and Kolar (1980) suggested that a clue to their reactivity is shown by the fact that any one of these compounds reacts with alkali to give diazomethane, and proposed that the hydrolytic formation of reactive methyl diazonium (Me-N_2^+) ions (23) (*Scheme 2.5*) occurs *in vivo*. From MNU (24) production is catalysed by OH⁻ and from MNNG (25) by cysteine or cysteinyl

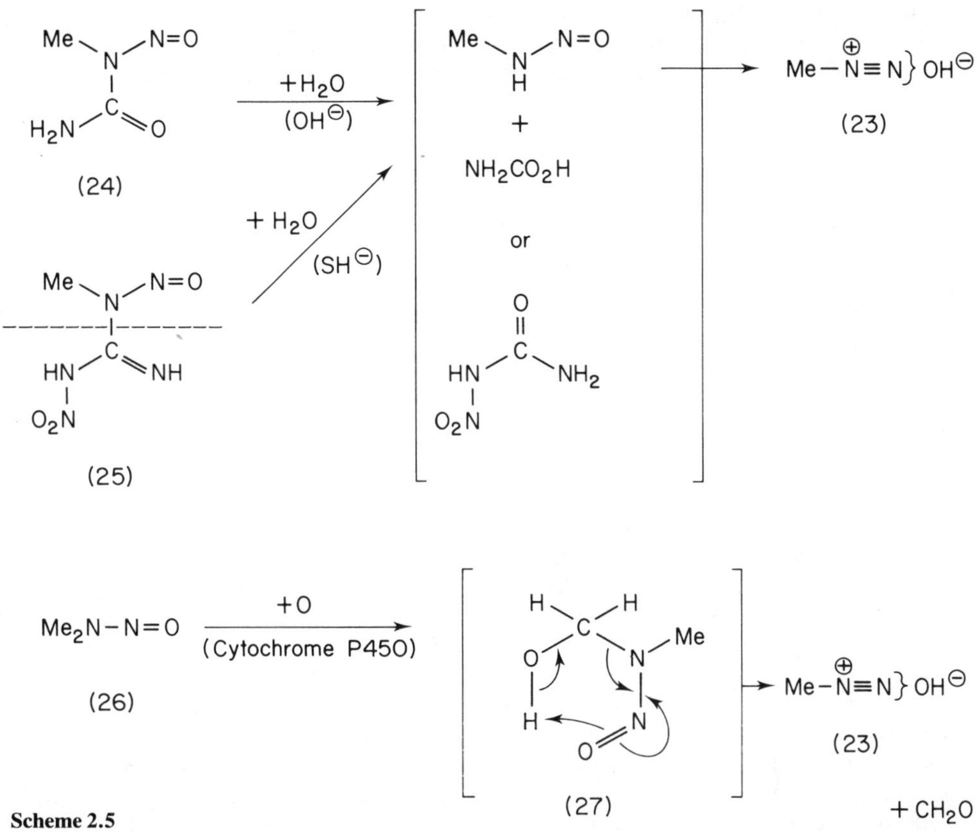

Scheme 2.5

peptides (Lawley and Thatcher, 1970). It might be said that the reactions concerned are non-enzymic chemical reactions (Hathway, 1980a), and that in these cases no metabolic activation is involved. Theoretically, alkylkation by agents which generate alkyldiazonium ions might be implemented through the alkyldiazonium cations *per se* or through the separate carbenium ions, but Hathway and Kolar (1980) consider that methylation is most likely to occur by a mechanism involving Me-N$_2^+$ cations rather than the well-known highly reactive species Me$^+$, used by the Millers (Miller, 1970; Miller and Miller, 1971). This observation (q.v.) agrees both with the conclusion of Friedman (1970) in Olah and von R. Schleyer's authoritative treatise and also with the result (Park, Archer and Wishnok, 1980) of feeding N,N-di-n-propylnitrosamine to rats, which produced 7-n-propylguanine but not 7-isopropylguanine, in the liver DNA, thus excluding carbo-cation participation.

In their discussion paper, Hathway and Kolar (1980) consider that in cytosol at pH 7.4, the energy-rich and very unstable Me-N$_2^+$ ions are in equilibrium with methanediazohydroxide (Eqn 2.1).

$$\text{Me-}\overset{+}{\text{N}}\equiv\text{N} + \text{H}_2\text{O} \rightleftharpoons \text{H}^+ + \text{Me-N=N-OH} \qquad (2.1)$$

and they noted that this would provide a source of carbo-cations only in strongly acidic, non-physiological medium (Moss, 1974). The ultimate carcinogenic form of the nitrosamide and nitrosamine (*see below*) agents is thus one of the electrophiles (Eqn 2.1), i.e. Me-N_2^+ or methanediazohydroxide. Hathway and Kolar (1980) considered that in competition with the faster loss of molecular nitrogen from Me-N_2^+ ions through the collapse of methanediazohydroxide (Eqn 2.1) to give methanol, the alkylation of nucleophilic sites in nucleic acid takes place by a reaction, which is described more correctly as S_N2, rather than as S_N1 as previously stated (Miller and Miller, 1971). The generation of Me-N_2^+ ions in close proximity to cellular DNA would, it was thought, result in the methylation of specific purine and pyrimidine nucleophilic sites through the formation of transient intermediates (Eqns 2.2 and 2.3). Whence the concomitant loss of molecular nitrogen and the collapse of the fugitive intermediates would transfer methyl groups to the oxygen and nitrogen nucleophiles (Eqns 2.4 and 2.5).

$$\text{Me--}\overset{+}{\text{N}}\equiv\text{N} + \text{ROH} \to \text{H}^+ + \text{Me--N=N--OR} \qquad (2.2)$$

$$\text{Me--}\overset{+}{\text{N}}\equiv\text{N} + \text{NHRR}' \to \text{H}^+ + \text{Me--N=N--NRR}' \qquad (2.3)$$

$$\text{Me--N=N--OR} \to \text{Me--OR} + N_2 \qquad (2.4)$$

$$\text{Me--N=N--NRR}' \to \text{Me--NRR}' + N_2 \qquad (2.5)$$

Good analogy exists for the various chemical reaction processes represented, for diazoethers have been isolated from other coupling reactions (Bücherer, 1909; Ginsberg and Goerdeler, 1961; Müller and Haiss, 1962), the coupling to nitrogen is very well known and, for example, MPT decomposes to give *N*-methylaniline (Kolar, 1980). It ought to be clearly stated here that essentially the whole of this argument applies also to the corresponding ethyl nitrosamides, *N*-ethyl-*N*-nitrosourea (ENU) and *N*-ethyl-*N*'-nitro-*N*-nitrosoguanidine (ENNG). Crucial experimental evidence is missing, however, and the underlying concept in this paragraph must be regarded as a reasonable or speculative chemical possibility. It would restore order (*see above*) to the great unifying principle of the Millers (Miller and Miller, 1971) who sought to match the nucleophilicity of genetic material that constitutes the probable receptors *in vivo* with the electrophilicity of the ultimate reactive forms of chemical carcinogens.

Product analysis sheds light on reactivity considerations and it is pertinent to follow the course of the reactions which have been suggested, from this point of view, but as the products, viz. the nucleoside analogues or 'adducts' obtained by breakdown of modified DNA, are associated with the question of reaction with cellular DNA, this matter will be discussed in Chapter 3.

In the case of *N*,*N*-dimethylnitrosamine (DMN) (26) [and of *N*,*N*-diethylnitrosamine (DEN)], the derivation of the reactive form (23) has been considered (Bartsch *et al.*, 1977) to proceed by elimination of the elements of formaldehyde from the cytochrome P450-mediated ω-oxidation product (27) via the cyclic mechanism that is represented (*Scheme 2.5*). As (26) has never been isolated, the mechanism operates in respect of a template reaction product. Since the pattern of DNA methylation products derived from DMN *in vivo* parallels that given by MNU (Chapter 3), this reflects a common mechanism of methylation via Me-N_2^+ ions, and the same supposition would be true for DEN and ENU with regard to Et-N_2^+ ions.

Hydrazines

Again, as in the case of DMN (*see above*), the derivation of the reactive form (23) of 1,2-dimethylhydrazine (*sym*-dimethylhydrazine) (28) (*Scheme 2.6*) has been

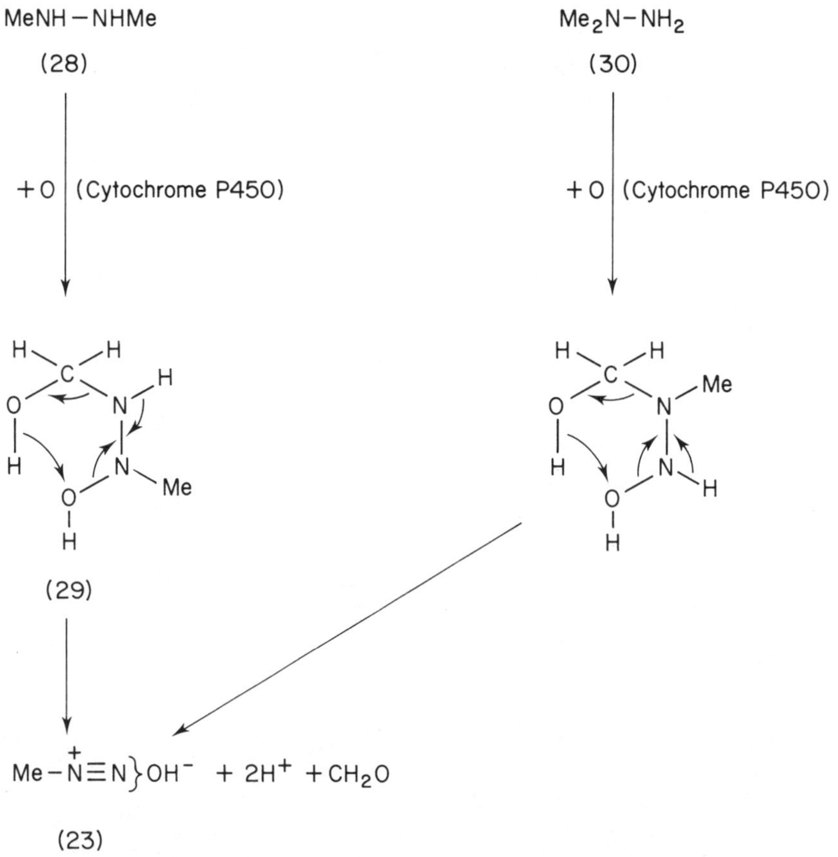

MeNH—NHMe   Me$_2$N—NH$_2$
   (28)   (30)

  +O │ (Cytochrome P450)   +O │ (Cytochrome P450)

[cyclic transition state structure (29)]   [cyclic transition state structure]

   (29)

Me—$\overset{+}{\text{N}}$≡N}OH$^-$ + 2H$^+$ + CH$_2$O

   (23)

Scheme 2.6

considered (Hathway, 1984b) to proceed by proton loss plus loss of the elements of formaldehyde from the cytochrome P450-mediated oxidation product (29) via the cyclic mechanism that is shown. As (29) is unstable and decomposes to give methane (Prough, 1973), the mechanism in question might be considered to take place in respect of a template reaction product. The pattern of DNA alkylation products *in vivo* parallels that afforded by DMN (Chapter 3), and this mirrors a common mechanism of methylation via Me-N$_2^+$ (23) (*Scheme 2.6*). Strictly similar considerations apply to 1,1-dimethylhydrazine (*asym*-dimethylhydrazine) (30), which also generates Me-N$_2^+$ ions (23) (*Scheme 2.6*). 1,2-Dimethylhydrazine was found to be carcinogenic in mice (Wiebecke *et al.*, 1969; Hawks, Farber and Magee, 1971/1972) and in rats (Druckrey *et al.*, 1967b; Preussman *et al.*, 1969) and 1,1-dimethylhydrazine was carcinogenic in mice after oral dosing (Roe, Grant and Millican, 1967; Toth, 1972, 1973).

The foregoing arguments would seem to infer that hydrazine would be non-carcinogenic, but other mechanisms of carcinogenicity are not ruled out. Despite its extensive manufacture (Raschig process), and its use in industrial chemical synthesis and as a fuel for fuel cells, there are no grounds for suspicion of carcinogenicity, and occupational exposure to hydrazine is unassociated with human cancer (Roe, 1978).

Phenyltriazenes

The same reactive form (23) would appear to be produced by elimination of the elements of formaldehyde from the cytochrome P450-mediated ω-oxidation product (32) (*Scheme 2.7*) of say 3,3-dimethyl-1-(2,4,6-trichlorophenyl)triazene (31) through the cyclic mechanism represented. It might be said in this context that (31) provides a further example (*see above*) where a particular metabolite [3-methyl-1-(2,4,6-trichlorophenyl)-2-triazeno]methyl β-D-glucuronide (33) (Kolar and Carubelli, 1979), formed in the liver, transports the mutagen (32), and facilitates its distribution throughout the body. The fact that no tissue fractions have greater enzyme activity for biotransformation of (31) into mutagen (32) than those of the liver, although more tumours are formed in some other organs than the liver, supports the foregoing transport mechanism (Bartsch *et al.*, 1977).

The new findings (q.v.) foreshadow the possible occurrence of a similarly constituted form for the transport of the well-established cancer chemotherapeutic agent, 5-(3,3-dimethyl-1-triazeno)imidazole-4-carboxamide, DIC or DTIC (34). Kolar, Maurer and Wildschütte (1980) have identified 5-(3-hydroxymethyl-3-methyl-1-triazeno)imidazole-4-carboxamide (35) as a urinary metabolite of (34) in rats, and they have confirmed the structure by synthesis.

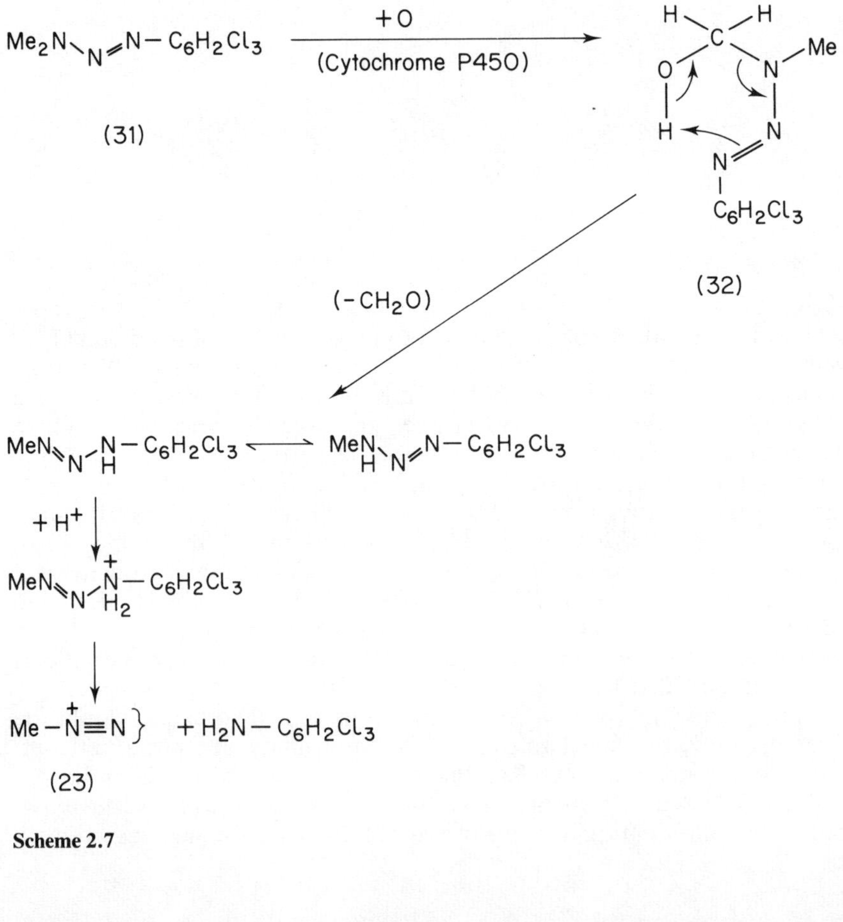

Scheme 2.7

Metals

Whilst it has long been suspected that chromium, nickel and cadmium are associated with industrial cancer, the reactive forms are largely unknown. In the case of chromium, however, Cr^{VI} has been found to be a mutagen in standard test systems (Venitt, 1974; Nishioka, 1975a,b; Petrilli and de Flora, 1977), whereas Cr^{3+} is non-mutagenic (Venitt, 1974; Petrilli and de Flora, 1977). Accordingly, it may be supposed that Cr^{VI} reacts with DNA, but since Cr^{VI} is transported across membranes whereas Cr^{3+} is not, the issue is not clearcut. Moreover, the significance of the recent finding (Goodgame, Hayman and Hathway, 1982) that Cr^{VI} reacts with ribonucleotides to give Cr^{V} is unknown. The basis for nickel carcinogenicity has not been investigated, and it would appear that soluble salts and complex ions of nickel have not been shown to be mutagenic in the Ames test but, for example, Ni_3S_2 causes lung tumours in animals and in man.

Vinyl chloride

There is a strong supposition (Van Duuren, 1975) that vinyl chloride (36) undergoes metabolic activation *in vivo* with the formation of chloroethylene oxide (37), which is transformed spontaneously (non-enzymic, chemical tautomerism) into chloroacetaldehyde (38) (Gross and Freiburg, 1969). Thus, there is plenty of supporting evidence (Barbin *et al.*, 1975; Bartsch and Montesano, 1975; Salmon, 1976) for vinyl chloride epoxidation *in vitro* by rat-liver cytochrome P450, and Göthe *et al.* (1974) have shown that when a cell-free preparation was exposed to (36) the reactive metabolite was trapped by 3,4-dichlorobenzenethiol in the form of 3,4-dichlorophenylthioacetaldehyde (mass spectrometry).

$$H_2C=CHCl \xrightarrow[\text{(Cytochrome P450)}]{(+O)} H_2C\underset{O}{-}CH-Cl \longleftrightarrow ClCH_2CH=O$$

(36)   (37)   (38)

CO$_2$H
|
CHCH$_2$SCH$_2$CH$_2$OH
|
NHAc

(39)

CO$_2$H
|
CHCH$_2$SCH$_2$CO$_2$H
|
NH$_2$

(40)

S(CH$_2$CO$_2$H)$_2$

(41)

The biological inter-relationship of glutathione *S*-epoxide transferase and substrate epoxide is well known, and the fact that (38) affords *in vivo* both *N*-acetyl-*S*-(2-hydroxyethyl)cysteine (39) and thiodiglycollic acid (41) (Green and Hathway, 1977), the principal metabolites of (36) (Green and Hathway, 1975, 1977), implies that (36) metabolism involves reaction between glutathione and (37) or (38). This is confirmed by the identification (mass fragmentometry) of *S*-(carboxymethyl)cysteine (30) amongst the hydrolytic products prepared from a hepatic extract from (36)-treated animals (Green and Hathway, 1977). Since (37) and (38) are mutagens in *S. typhimurium* strains (Bartsch, Malaveille and Montesano, 1975; McCann *et al.*, 1975a; Malaveille *et al.*, 1975) and in Chinese hamster V79 cells (Huberman, Bartsch and Sachs, 1975), both of these substances may contribute to (36) carcinogenicity in mammals.

The fact that the same nucleoside analogues, viz. 9-(β-D-2'-deoxyribofuranosyl)imidazo[2,1-*i*]purine (etheno-dA) and 1-(β-D-2'-deoxyribofuranosyl)imidazo[1,2-*c*]pyrimidin-2[1H]-one(etheno-dC) (Chapter 3) are both formed *in vitro* by interaction of (38) or (37) with calf-thymus DNA and in the liver DNA of rats exposed chronically to (36) in their drinking water (Green and Hathway, 1978) provides proof of the modification of target-organ DNA by (36) and implies a common mechanism both *in vitro* and *in vivo*. In both cases, formation of chloroethylene oxide (37) is involved, followed by initial (S$_N$2) alkylation.

Since vinyl bromide and vinyl chloride (36) alkylate nucleic acid similarly (Ottenwaelder, Laib and Bolt, 1979), the metabolic activation that was established in the case of (36) applies also to the bromide analogue. It will be appreciated that

$$\text{BrCH}_2\text{CH}_2\text{Br} \xrightarrow{(+O)} \underset{\underset{\text{OH}}{|}}{\text{BrCH}_2\text{CHBr}} \xrightarrow{(-\text{HBr})} \underset{\underset{O}{\|}}{\text{BrCH}_2\text{CH}}$$

(42)   (43)

the mechanism of conversion of compound (36) to compound (38) in the activation and carcinogenicity of (36) can be extended to other industrial chemicals. Thus, imidazocyclization of DNA purine and pyrimidine residues attributable to vinyl chloride-related (37) and (38) (Chapter 3) would account both for the covalent binding to tissue DNA of the bromoacetaldehyde (43) metabolite of 1,2-dibromoethane (42) (Hill et al., 1978) and for the associated (42) mutagenicity (Malling and de Serres, 1969; Ames, 1971; Buselmaier, Röhrborn and Propping, 1973; Cumming and Walton, 1973; Brem, Stein and Rosenkranz, 1974) and (42) carcinogenicity in rodents (Olson et al., 1973; Government Report Announcements Index, 1979). Under the conditions of the NCI bioassay, 1,2-dichloroethane was found also to be carcinogenic in rodents (Bahlman et al., 1978; Department of Health, Welfare and Education, 1978; Government Report Announcements Index, 1978). Metabolic study (Rannug and Bëye, 1979) showed the bile of treated animals to contain mutagen(s) 15–30 min after dosing, but 2-chloroethanol proved to be a non-mutagen. The results support the metabolic activation of 1,2-dihalogenoethanes through conjugation with glutathione. In the case, *N*-acetyl-*S*-(2-chloroethyl)-L-cysteine and *S*-(2-chloroethyl)-L-cysteine (44) caused base-pair substitution mutagenicity in *S. typhimurium* TA1535 strain. There is thus a remarkable similarity between (36) metabolism (Green and Hathway, 1975, 1977) and that of the 1,2-dihalogenoethanes (q.v.).

$$\underset{\underset{\text{NH(Ac)}}{|}}{\overset{\overset{\text{CO}_2\text{H}}{|}}{\text{CHCH}_2\text{SCH}_2\text{CH}_2\text{Cl}}}$$

(44)

Polycyclic aromatic hydrocarbons

Boyland (1950) suggested the intermediacy of epoxides to account for the metabolism of naphthalene, anthracene, phenanthrene etc. in mammals into *trans*-dihydrodiols, and it was found later that the carcinogenic and more complicated polycyclic aromatic hydrocarbons were metabolized by liver microsomal enzymes into *trans*-dihydrodiols. In these cases, as well, there was a considerable body of evidence for intermediate epoxide formation (Sims and Grover, 1974). Discussion of the metabolism of a single polycyclic aromatic hydrocarbon, for example benzo[a]pyrene (45), which was referred to in the previous section of this chapter, will serve to illustrate the metabolic activation of this series of compounds. Compound (45) affords three (−)*trans*-dihydrodiols, viz. the 4,5- (46), 7,8- (47) and 9,10-*trans*-dihydrodiols (48) (Yang and Gelboin, 1976), besides various phenols and quinones. It is germane that (46) is formed at the high electron density 'K region' of the molecule (Daudel and Pullman, 1945) that is

32 *Activation of chemical carcinogens in the mammal*

equivalent to an activated phenanthrene double bond, which Robinson (1946) considered characterized most carcinogenic polycyclic aromatic hydrocarbons. In the cyclohexane ring in which the hydroxyls are substituted, (47) and (48) possess, however, an olefinic bond capable of further epoxidation (Booth and Sims, 1974). The resulting 'bay-region' 7,8-diol-9,10-epoxide (49) is formed in relatively high yield compared with that of the 9,10-diol-7,8-epoxide (50). 'Bay-region' epoxides are ones where the epoxide group is adjacent to the bay lying between an angular benzo group and the rest of the molecule (Jerina and Daly, 1977). From molecular-orbital calculations, Jerina and Lehr (1977) have predicted that the 'bay-region' diol-epoxide, for example (49), is the most chemically reactive of all of the possible diol-epoxides which can be derived from any one polycyclic aromatic hydrocarbon, for example (45).

It is interesting that diol-epoxides occur in two stereoisomeric forms, viz. the *syn*-isomer (51) where the epoxide is on the same side of the cyclohexane ring as the benzilic hydroxyl, and the *anti*-isomer (52) where it is on the opposite side. As *trans*-dihydrodiols can occur as (+) and (−)-optical enantiomers, four isomeric forms are possible of each diol-epoxide, i.e. one *syn*- and one *anti*- form of each optically active enantiomer. All four isomers of some 'bay-region' diol-epoxides have been synthesized (Yagi et al., 1977) and the (+)*anti*-7,8-dihydrodiol-9,10-epoxide of benzo[a]pyrene (45) is considered to be the most biologically potent (Slaga et al., 1979). It is also known that the most chemically active epoxides are not the most mutagenic/carcinogenic. The *syn*-epoxides are, of course, more reactive than the *anti*-isomers.

In the case of the highly carcinogenic 7,12-dimethylbenz[a]anthracene (53), metabolic attack occurs also at the methyl C-atoms, giving sequential formation of hydroxy compounds, aldehydes and carboxylic acids. The sulphate conjugates of the hydroxy compounds, which are themselves reactive benzilic esters, show high carcinogenic potential and would, therefore, contribute directly to the expression of (53) carcinogenicity.

Microbiological products

Aflatoxins

The structure of the nucleoside adducts (Chapter 3) resulting from the hydrolysis of salmon-sperm DNA and rat-liver ribosomal RNA, which had been modified by aflatoxin B_1 (54) in the presence, respectively, of rat and hamster-liver microsomes, is consistent with the interaction of aflatoxin B_1 2,3-epoxide (55) (Lin, Miller and Miller, 1977). Epoxide formation in this regard is supported by the fact that (*a*) biochemical study (Lin et al., 1978) has shown 2,3-dihydro-2,3-dihydroxyaflatoxin-B_1 (56) to be a major metabolite of (54) *in vitro*, and (*b*) that a negligible amount of compound (56) was formed from compound (54) in the presence of DNA, under

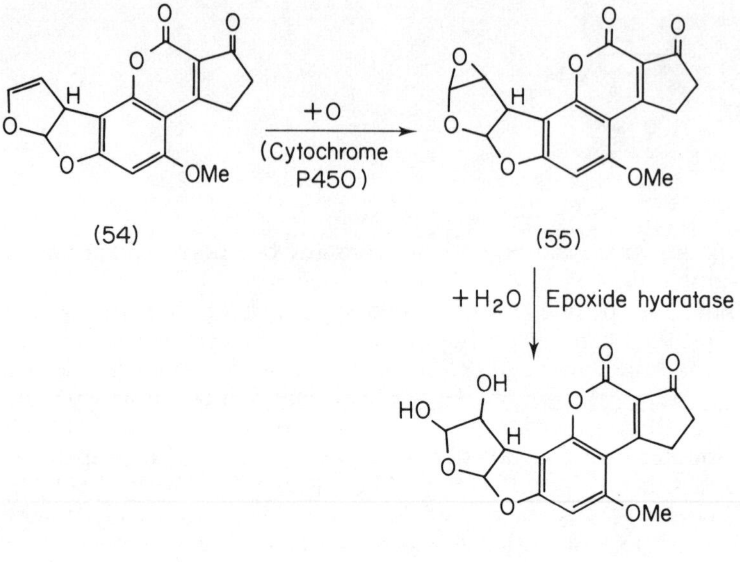

(54) → (55)

+O
(Cytochrome P450)

+H₂O | Epoxide hydratase
↓

(56)

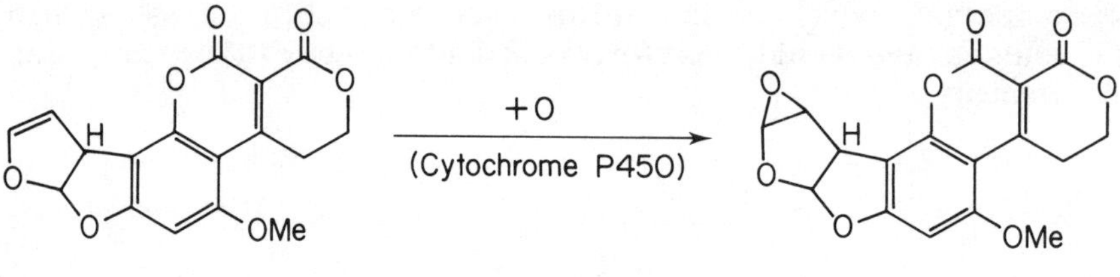

(57) → (58)

+O
(Cytochrome P450)

the same conditions as those operating for (*a*). Evidence resulting from essentially similar studies made with aflatoxin G₁ (57) (Garner *et al.*, 1979) to those made with (54) (Lin, Miller and Miller, 1977; Lin *et al.*, 1978) showed the 2,3-epoxide (58) to be the putative reactive metabolite in this case as well.

Plant products

Cycasin

The mutagenic and carcinogenic properties of cycasin (59) and other methylazoxy methanol (60) derivatives (Magee, Montesano and Preussmann, 1976; Montesano and Bartsch, 1978) closely resemble those of the nitrosamines (*see above*), and evidence for the methylation of rat-brain (Nagata and Matsumoto, 1969) and liver

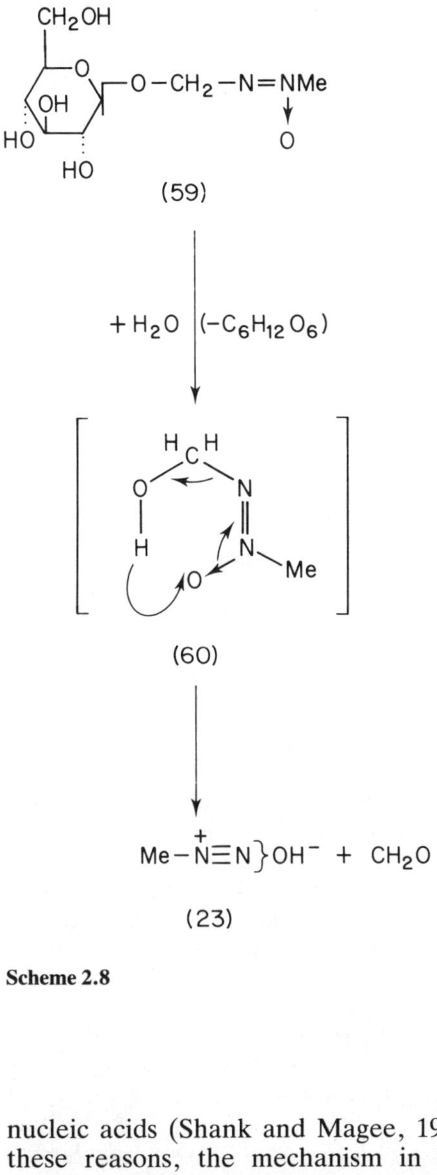

Scheme 2.8

nucleic acids (Shank and Magee, 1967) *in vivo* was found 15–20 years ago. For these reasons, the mechanism in the accompanying scheme (*Scheme 2.8*) is proposed (Hathway, 1984a) to account for the reactivity of (59) and (60).

Safrole

Whilst epoxidation of the hepatocarcinogen, safrole (61) occurs *in vitro*, furnishing 1'-hydroxysafrole-2',3'-oxide (63) (Stillwell *et al.*, 1974), compound (61) is metabolized in rodents into 1'-hydroxysafrole (62). Safrole-1'-sulphate (64), which is a benzilic ester, has been identified (Wislocki *et al.*, 1976) as the ultimate reactive metabolite of (61), responsible for carcinogenicity of (61) in mammals.

36 Activation of chemical carcinogens in the mammal

[Structures (61) → (62); (62) → (63); (61) → (64)]

(61) benzo[1,3]dioxole-CH₂-CH=CH₂

(62) benzo[1,3]dioxole-CH(OH)-CH=CH₂

(63) benzo[1,3]dioxole-CH(OH)-CH-CH₂ (epoxide)

(64) benzo[1,3]dioxole-CH(O-SO₃H)-CH=CH₂

Biosynthesis of reactive metabolites and matching tissue specificities

The significance of the production of reactive metabolites of carcinogens *in vivo* depends on its accountability for the known tissue specificities. Logically, this subject ought to be considered at this stage in the narrative, but arguments dealing with product analysis (Chapter 3) and DNA repair (Chapter 4), which are cogent, cannot be treated as adequately as they may merit. It is feasible, however, to cite some limitations to the production of reactive metabolites *de novo* and, thus, to indicate to some extent the possible scope of the cancer process. This section of the chapter is concerned with these considerations.

To recapitulate the β-naphthylamine story, N-hydroxylation occurs in the liver and, in dogs and monkeys and in man, the mutagen is converted immediately by the hepatic cytosol into the *N*-glucuronide (*see above*), which is transported to the bladder, where it is deconjugated by the lumen epithelial cells, and where tumours are induced. In mice, which are deficient in UDPGT, 2-naphthylhydroxylamine (which was synthesized in the liver) provokes hepatoma induction. Cats, rabbits and rats, which lack the mixed functional oxidase for effecting N-hydroxylation, are resistant to β-naphthylamine.

An arylhydroxylamine might be activated further *in vivo* by esterification, as the energy required for elimination of the elements of acid in order to generate reactive electrophiles is less than that necessary for the elimination of the elements of water from the parent arylhydroxylamine. Thus, sulphation is implemented by soluble liver sulphotransferase systems and, in some cases, a deficiency of this enzyme can confer resistance to carcinogenesis. Sulphation is not, however, the only mechanism available for activation, and the absence of this enzyme system from a tissue does not necessarily preclude carcinogenesis. For example, rat ear-duct and mammary glands are very low in sulphotransferase activity, but they are tissue sensitive to 2AAF tumours (Irving, Janss and Russell, 1971). These tissues may have some other activating system like acetyl transferase or peroxidase, which will generate a reactive ester form, but alternatively ring–chain tautomerism (*Scheme 2.4*) may be relevant. But, in the case of β-naphthylamine, esterification is irrelevant to metabolic activation, as, for example, the chronic administration of 2-acetnaphthalide to dogs for 2 years did not induce tumours, whereas the equivalent dose of the parent β-naphthylamine, given in the same way, produced bladder cancer in all of the animals exposed (Conzelman and Flanders, 1972). 2-Naphthylhydroxylamine is, therefore, the ultimate carcinogen *per se*, at any rate in dogs, in the case of β-naphthylamine. Although rabbits are resistant to 2AAF liver cancer, they develop bladder tumours, presumably also via unesterified arylhydroxylamine.

Benzidine bladder cancer requires a transport form, presumably a glucuronide for an *N*-hydroxy compound, because (*a*) *N*-acetylbenzidine was transformed by fortified liver microsomes to give *N*-hydroxy-*N,N'*-diacetylbenzidine plus 3-hydroxy-*N,N'*-diacetylbenzidine and, in the living animal, pre-treatment with 3-methylcholanthrene enhanced both N- and 3-hydroxylations, (*b*) *N*-hydroxy-*N,N'*-diacetylbenzidine bound to RNA involving liver cytosol *N,O*-acyltransferase, and (*c*) *N*-hydroxy-*N,N'*-diacetylbenzidine was mutagenic in *S. typhimurium* TA1538 strain (Morton, King and Baetcke, 1979).

In rats, there is a good correlation between organ-specific *N*-nitrosamine tumours (Druckrey *et al.*, 1967a) and the enzymic capacity of the relevant organs to form reactive metabolites (Montesano and Bartsch, 1976). Tumour incidence increases in the order c.n.s. < bladder < forestomach < kidneys < respiratory tract < nasal cavities < oesophagus < liver, and this was followed by formation of O^6-methylguanine in the DNA of those tissues (Chapter 3) and its persistence there (Chapter 4). There would appear, however, to be, in the various tissues, a balance between the activities of activating enzyme systems and the ones responsible for detoxifying reactive metabolites, and this would account for the induction of (or resistance to) tumours. Thus, in connection with *N*-nitrosamine liver tumours, the inhibition of the hepatic drug-metabolizing enzymes is paralleled by a diminished incidence (of tumours), although, in many circumstances, there is an accompanying increase in the incidence of tumours in other parts of the body.

High sensitivity of the fibroblastic elements tends to interfere with the potential response of (liver) parenchymatous tissue, where the hepatocarcinogen is administered systematically, and animals often succumb to rapidly growing sarcomas before the specialized tissue has had time to respond (Berenblum, 1974). These conclusions were reached from the carcinogenicity testing of amino-azo dyes (Berenblum, 1974), and the case of vinyl chloride liver cancer would seem to be unexceptional. Thus, in the chronic situation where administered to experimental animals either by inhalation or by injection, it caused angiosarcoma of the liver (Maltoni and Lefemine, 1974a,b, 1975; Maltoni, 1977a). In contrast to hepatic fibroblastic DNA, hepatocyte DNA (in the parenteral administrations) is protected by the high activity of the powerful glutathione, glutathione *S*-epoxide transferase detoxifying enzyme system from attack by the vinyl chloride-related mutagens, chloroethylene oxide and chloroacetaldehyde (*see above*). But, where high concentrations of vinyl chloride reach the liver as, for example, by enteral dosing, transformation into mutagenic chloroethylene oxide in the hepatocytes would tend to occur in sufficient amounts to overcome the defence mechanism (q.v.) there. In the case of parenteral exposure, the chloroacetaldehyde rearrangement product has a $t_{0.5}$ value which is long enough to enable reaction with hepatic fibroblastic DNA. Berenblum (1974) says that, at lower oral dose-levels, hepatocarcinogens produce mixed sarcomas and hepatomas.

With regard to polycyclic aromatic hydrocarbons, benzo[a]pyrene is metabolized into dihydrodiols by several mammalian tissues through the successive action of cytochrome P450 and epoxide hydratase. These tissues include rat colon, liver and lung and human colon, liver, lung and lymphocytes. Metabolic study of a number of polycyclic aromatic hydrocarbons by mouse skin, a target tissue for polycyclic aromatic hydrocarbons, shows all of the compounds to be converted into dihydrodiols, but the relative proportions formed differ from those by rat-liver subcellular components and contain more dihydrodiols which yield bay-region diol-epoxides. Cultures of human bronchus, like mouse skin, afford DNA and RNA adducts of benzo[a]pyrene, via the *anti*-isomer of the 7,8-dihydrodiol-9,10-epoxides (Phillips and Sims, 1979). Wide distribution of epoxide hydratase and glutathione transferase is shown by the epoxide hydratase activities of mouse, rat and human skin (Oesch, Schmassmann and Bentley, 1978) and by the fact that glutathione conjugates are produced by benzo[a]pyrene metabolism in cultures of human colon, and by several other tissues (Autrup, 1979).

Finally, Hathway (1980b) has suggested a spillover model for enzymic reactions under limiting conditions, and where an alternative metabolic pathway is potentially available. Thus, the identification in mice, in which 1,1,2-trichloroethylene (65) is both mutagenic and tumorogenic, of the (65) metabolites, trichloroacetic acid (68), trichloroethanol glucuronide (69) and dichloroacetic acid (71), implied rearrangement of 1,1,2-trichloroethylene oxide (66) into both chloral

$Cl_2C=CH_2$

(72)

$+ O$ | (Cytochrome P450)

$ClC\overset{Cl}{\underset{O}{-}}CH_2 \longleftrightarrow ClCCH_2Cl$
$\overset{\|}{O}$

(73)

(67) and dichloroacetyl chloride (70) (Hathway, 1980b). By analogy with vinylidene chloride (1,1-dichloroethylene) (72), where there was corresponding formation of chloroacetyl chloride (73) (Jones and Hathway, 1978a) and the binding to mouse-kidney DNA (Hathway, 1977; Jones and Hathway, 1978b), the formation of (70) appears to be consistent with (65)-induced murine liver cancer (Lloyd, Moore and Breslin, 1975; IARC, 1976; American Conference of Government Industrial Hygienists, 1978). The idea of a spillover model for a biological situation, where there is a massive excess of the substrate (66), relative to catalytic sites for the usual rearrangement under physiological conditions into compound (67) (Hathway, 1980b), is consistent with the small proportion of compound (71) in relation to the large one of compound (68) which is eliminated in the urine of treated mice. In the case exemplified here, an alternative metabolic pathway for compound (65) is followed in mice, but not in rats and in man (Jones and Hathway, 1978b), to an extent that is commensurate with liver-tumour induction.

A spillover model may be applicable to Dichlorvos, O,O-dimethyl-2,2-dichlorovinyl phosphate (74) (*Scheme 2.9*) mutagenicity (Cahere *et al.*, 1978) and possible murine carcinogenicity (IARC, 1979), which otherwise affords (Casida, McBride and Niedermeier, 1962; Hodgson and Casida, 1962; Hutson *et al.*, 1971) innocuous products (*Scheme 2.9*). Under limiting conditions, such as high chronic dosage of (74), the product (76) of the phosphate hydrolysis of O-methyl-2,2-dichlorovinyl phosphate (75) would generate highly reactive dichloroacetaldehyde (77). Löfroth (1978) has shown that (77) yields a stronger response than (74) in the Ames test, and thus would account for the mutagenicity of (74) observed (Cahere *et al.*, 1978).

The catabolism of endogenous methacrylic acid (78) (*Scheme 2.10*) gives acetate and CO_2, and this metabolic pathway is followed by the compound (78), which is produced from relatively large doses of exogenous methyl methacrylate (Bratt and Hathway, 1977). Small amounts of methylmalonate, succinate, β-hydroxyisobutyrate (79) and 2-formylpropionate (80) were also detected in this tracer study. If the occurrence of transplacental haemangiomas in the rat pups of dams, treated systemically with methyl methacrylate on days 5, 10 and 15 of gestation (Singh, Lawrence and Autian, 1972) is significant, however, it may be necessary to enlist a spillover model for the high substrate to key enzyme situation. Formation of mutagenic epoxide and a lack of detoxifying epoxide hydratase and

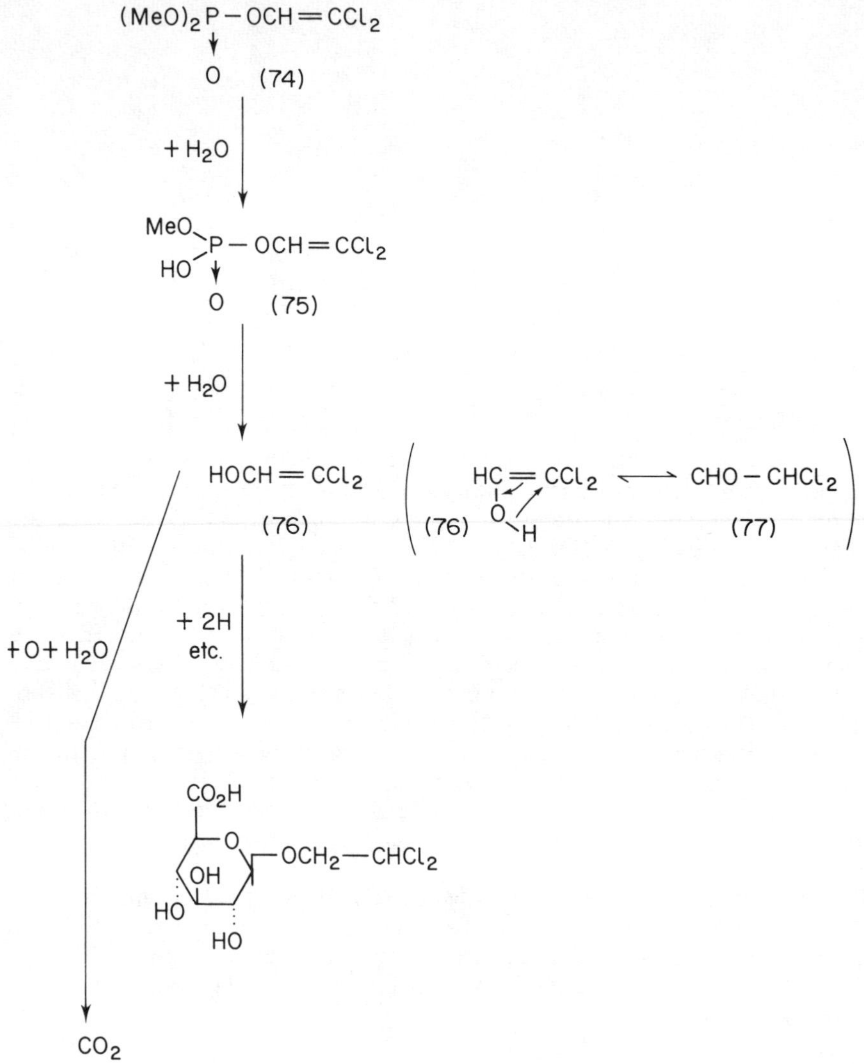

Scheme 2.9

$(MeO)_2P(=O)-OCH=CCl_2$ (74)

$+H_2O$ ↓

$MeO-P(OH)(=O)-OCH=CCl_2$ (75)

$+H_2O$ ↓

$HOCH=CCl_2$ (76) $\left(HC\underset{O-H}{=\!=\!=}CCl_2 \;\;(76) \longleftrightarrow CHO-CHCl_2 \;\;(77) \right)$

$+O+H_2O$ / $+2H$ etc. ↓

[glucuronide: CO_2H, OH, HO, HO on pyranose ring]—OCH_2-CHCl_2

↓

CO_2

glutathione, glutathione S-epoxide transferase activity in the fetal livers at those times in gestation may account for Singh, Lawrence and Autian's observation, but intraperitoneal injection of the pregnant dams is open to suspicion, and is not used in straightforward teratogenicity testing.

Whilst, undoubtedly, spillover models have wide application, it is relevant that biotransformations, however attractive, do not take place outside a system regulated by the physiological conditions, and in which only kinetically controlled biochemical and chemical reactions for the disposal of a foreign compound are followed.

In conclusion, a critical balance between the activities of the activating enzyme systems and those of the detoxifying processes seems to determine the sensitivity

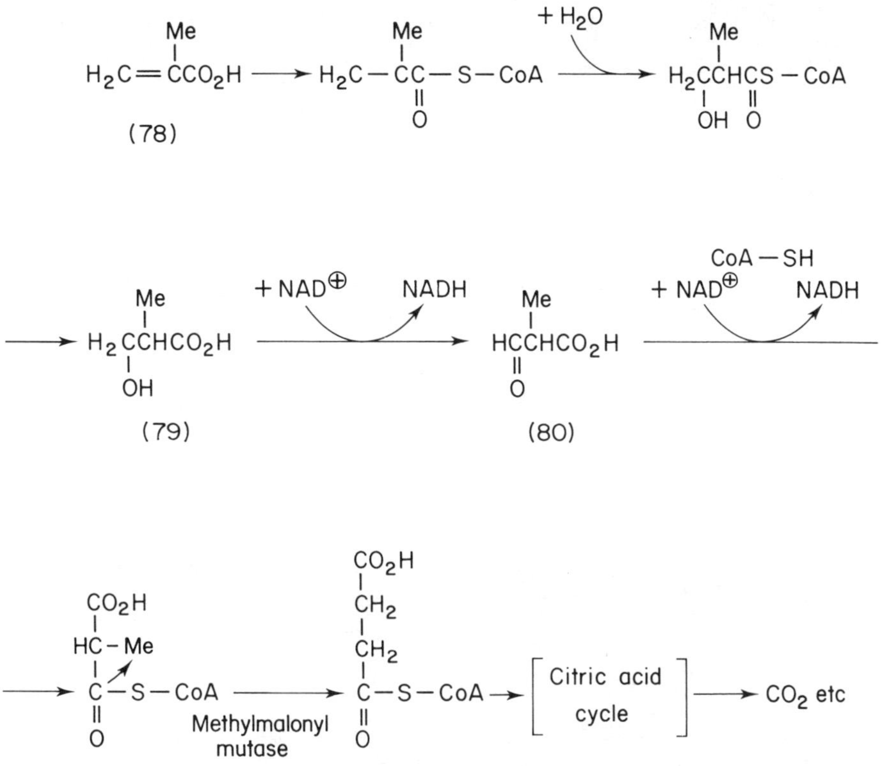

Scheme 2.10

shown by the various tissues to attack by any particular chemical carcinogen. Supporting evidence will be given by the modification of nucleic acids (Chapter 3) and the persistence of nucleoside analogues in target-tissue nucleic acid (Chapter 4). An interaction between cell replication and tissue-specific DNA-repair processes must contribute, in the ultimate analysis, to the expression of carcinogenicity. But in general, there is broad agreement between the biochemical evidence, discussed in the final section of this chapter, and tissue specificity.

Bibliography and references

ALBERT, Z. (1956) *Arch. Immunol. Ter. Dosw.*, **4**, 189
AMERICAN CONFERENCE OF GOVERNMENT INDUSTRIAL HYGIENISTS (1978) *Threshold Limit Values for Chemical Substances and Physical Agents in the Workroom Environment with Intended Changes for 1977.* pp. 40, 41
AMES, B.N. (1971) In *Chemical Mutagens: Principles and Methods for their Detection.* Ed. A. Hollaender. Vol. 1. pp. 267–281. New York: Plenum Press
AMES, B.N. (1972) In *Mutagenic Effects of Environmental Contaminants.* Eds E. Sutton and M. Harris. pp. 57–66. New York: Academic Press
AMES, B.N., DURSTON, W.E., YAMASAKI, E. and LEE, F.D. (1973) *Proc. Natl Acad. Sci. USA*, **70**, 2281
AMES, B.N., GURNEY, E.G., MILLER, J.A. and BARTSCH, H. (1972) *Proc. Natl Acad. Sci. USA*, **69**, 3128
AMES, B.N., KAMMEN, H.O. and YAMASAKI, E. (1975) *Proc. Natl Acad. Sci. USA*, **72**, 2423

AMES, B.N., LEE, F.D. and DURSTON, W.E. (1973) *Proc. Natl Acad. Sci. USA*, **70**, 782
AMES, B.N., McCANN, J. and YAMASAKI, E. (1975) *Mutat. Res.*, **31**, 347
AMES, B.N., SIMS, P. and GROVER, P.L. (1972) *Science*, **176**, 47
AUTRUP, H. (1979) *Biochem. Pharmacol.*, **28**, 1727
BAETJER, A.M. (1950) *Arch. Ind. Hyg.*, **2**, 505
BAHLMAN, L.J., LEIDEL, N.A., PARKER, J.C., STEIN, H.P., THOMAS, A.W., WOOLF, B.S. et al. (1978) *Am. Ind. Hyg. Assoc. J.*, **39**, A35, A37, A39, A41, A43
BAKER, J.W. (1934) *Tautomerism*, pp. 173–200. London: George Routledge & Sons
BARBIN, A., BRESIL, H., CROISY, A., JACQUIGNON, P., MALAVEILLE, C., MONTESANO, R. et al. (1975) *Biochem. Biophys. Res. Commun.*, **67**, 596
BARTSCH, H., MALAVEILLE, C. and MONTESANO, R. (1975) *Int. J. Cancer*, **14**, 429
BARTSCH, H., MALAVEILLE, C. and MONTESANO, R. (1976) In *Screening Tests in Chemical Carcinogenesis*. Eds R. Montesano, H. Bartsch and L. Tomatis. pp. 467–486. Lyon, France: IARC
BARTSCH, H., MARGINSON, G.P., MALAVEILLE, C., CAMUS, A.M., BRUN, G., MARGINSON, J.M. et al. (1977) *Arch. Toxikol.*, **39**, 51
BARTSCH, H. and MONTESANO, R. (1975) *Mutat. Res.*, **32**, 93
BERENBLUM, I. (1974) *Carcinogenesis as a Biological Problem*. pp. 12, 16. Amsterdam: North-Holland Publishing Company
BIDSTRUP, P.L. and CASE, R.A.M. (1956) *Br. J. Ind. Med.*, **13**, 260
BLOCH, B. and DREIFUSS, W. (1921) *Schweiz. med. Wochenschr.*, **51**, 1033
BONSER, G.M. (1943) *J. Pathol. Bacteriol.*, **55**, 1
BONSER, G.M., BOYLAND, E., BUSBY, E.R., CLAYSON, D.B., GROVER, P.L. and JULL, J.W. (1963) *Br. J. Cancer*, **17**, 127
BONSER, G.M., CLAYSON, D.B., JULL, J.W. and PYRAH, L.N. (1956) *Br. J. Cancer*, **10**, 533
BONSER, G.M. and JULL, J.W. (1956) *J. Pathol. Bacteriol.*, **72**, 489
BOOTH, J. and SIMS, P. (1974) *FEBS Lett.*, **47**, 30
BOYLAND, E. (1950) *Biochem. Soc. Symp.* No. 5, pp. 40–54
BOYLAND, E., MANSON, D. and ORR, S.F.D. (1957) *Biochem. J.*, **65**, 417
BRATT, H. and HATHWAY, D.E. (1977) *Br. J. Cancer*, **36**, 114
BREM, H., STEIN, A.G. and ROSENKRANZ, H.S. (1974) *Cancer Res.*, **34**, 2576
BRINTON, H.P., FRASIER, E.S. and KOVEN, A.L. (1952) *Publ. Health Rep. Wash.*, **67**, 835
BROWN, D.V. and NORLIND, L.M. (1959) *Am. J. Pathol.*, **35**, 696
BROWN, D.V. and NORLIND, L.M. (1961) *Arch. Pathol.*, **72**, 251
BRYAN, G.T., BROWN, R.R. and PRICE, J.M. (1964) *Cancer Res.*, **24**, 596
BÜCHERER, H.T. (1909) *Ber. Dtsch Chem. Ges.*, **42**, 47
BUSELMAIER, W., RÖHRBORN, G. and PROPPING, P. (1973) *Mutat. Res.*, **21**, 25
CAHERE, A., ORTALI, V.A., CARDAMONE, G. and MORPURGO, G. (1978) *Chem.-Biol. Interact.*, **22**, 297
CASE, R.A.M., HOSKER, M.E., McDONALD, D.B. and PEARSON, J.T. (1954) *Br. J. Ind. Med.*, **11**, 75
CASIDA, J.E., McBRIDE, L. and NIEDERMEIER, R.P. (1962) *J. Agric. Food Chem.*, **10**, 370
CHIEF INSPECTOR OF FACTORIES (1933) *Ann. Rep. Chief Inspector of Factories for the Year 1932.* p. 103. London: HMSO
CHIEF INSPECTOR OF FACTORIES (1952) *Ann. Rep. Chief Inspector of Factories for the Year 1950.* p. 145. London: HMSO
CLAYSON, D.B. (1962) *Chemical Carcinogenesis*. London: J & A Churchill
CLAYSON, D.B. (1974) *J. Natl Cancer Inst.*, **52**, 1685
CLAYSON, D.B. (1975) In *Biology of Cancer*, 2nd edn. Eds E.J. Ambrose and F.J.C. Roe. pp. 163–179. Chichester: Ellis Horwood
CLAYSON, D.B. and COOPER, E.H. (1970) *Adv. Cancer Res.*, **13**, 271
CLAYSON, D.B. and PRINGLE, J.A.S. (1961) *Br. J. Cancer*, **20**, 564
COMMONER, B., VITHAYATHIL, A.J. and HENRY, J.I. (1974) *Nature*, **249**, 850
CONROW, R.B. and BERNSTEIN, S. (1971) *J. Org. Chem.*, **36**, 863
CONZELMAN, G.M. and FLANDERS, L.E. (1972) *Proc. West Pharmacol. Soc.*, **15**, 96
COOK, J.W., HEWETT, C.L. and HIEGER, I. (1933) *J. Chem. Soc.*, p. 395
CRAMER, J.W., MILLER, J.A. and MILLER, E.C. (1960) *J. Biol. Chem.*, **235**, 885
CUMMING, R.B. and WALTON, M.F. (1973) *Food Cosmet. Toxicol.*, **11**, 547
DAUDEL, R. and PULLMAN, A. (1945) *C.R. Hebd. Séances Acad. Sci., Paris*, **220**, 888
DE BAUN, J.R., MILLER, E.C. and MILLER, J.A. (1970) *Cancer Res.*, **30**, 577
DE BAUN, J.R., ROWLEY, J.Y., MILLER, E.C. and MILLER, J.A. (1968) *Proc. Soc. Exp. Biol. Med.*, **129**, 268
DEICHMANN, W.B. and RADOMSKI, J.L. (1969) *J. Natl Cancer Inst.*, **43**, 263
DEPARTMENT OF HEALTH, EDUCATION AND WELFARE (1978) *1,2-Dichloroethane.* Current Intelligence Bulletin. DHEW (NIOSH) Publ., pp. 78–149

DOLL, R. (1958) *Br. J. Ind. Med.*, **15**, 217
DOLL, R., MORGAN, L.G. and SPEIZER, F.E. (1970) *Br. J. Cancer*, **24**, 623
DRUCKREY, H. (1943) *Klin. Wochenschr.*, **22**, 532
DRUCKREY, H. (1951) *Arzneimittel-Forschung*, **1**, 383
DRUCKREY, H. (1959) In *Chemical Carcinogenesis: Mechanism of Action*. Ciba Colloq. pp. 110–130. London: Churchill
DRUCKREY, H. and KÜPFMÜLLER, K. (1948) *Z. Naturforschung*, **3B**, 254
DRUCKREY, H. and KÜPFMÜLLER, K. (1949) *Dosis und Wirkung*. Aulendorf-im-Württemberg: Editio Cantor
DRUCKREY, H., PREUSSMANN, R., IVANKOVIC, S. and SCHMÄHL, D. (1967a) *Z. Krebsforschung*, **69**, 103
DRUCKREY, H., PREUSSMANN, R., MATZKIES, F. and IVANKOVIC, S. (1967b) *Nátúrwissenschaften*, **54**, 285
DRUCKREY, H. and SCHMÄHL, D. (1962) *Nátúrwissenschaften*, **49**, 217
DRUCKREY, H., STEINHOFF, D., BEUTHNER, H., SCHNEIDER, H. and KLÄRNER, P. (1963) *Arzneimittel-Forschung*, **13**, 320
DURSTON, W.E. and AMES, B.N. (1974) *Proc. Natl Acad. Sci. USA*, **71**, 737
DYBING, E. and SOEDERLUND, E.J. (1978) In *Proceedings of the Symposium on Conjugation Reactions in Drug Biotransformations*. Ed. A. Aitio. pp. 283–292. Amsterdam: Elsevier
DYBING, E., SOEDERLUND, E.J. and HAUG, L.T. (1979) *Cancer Res.*, **39**, 3268
DYBING, E., VON BAHR, C., AUNE, T., GLAUMANN, H., LEVITT, D.S. and THORGEIRSSON, S.S. (1979) *Cancer Res.*, **39**, 4206
ENGEL, H. (1920) *Gewerbehyg. Unfallverhüt.*, **8**, 81
FELLER, D.R., MORITA, M. and GILLETTE, J.R. (1971) *Proc. Soc. Exp. Biol. Med.*, **137**, 433
FRIEDMAN, L. (1970) In *Carbonium Ions*. Eds G.A. Olah and P. von R. Schleyer. Vol. 2. pp. 655–711. New York: John Wiley and Sons
GARNER, R.C., MARTIN, C.N., SMITH, J.R.L., COLES, B.F. and TOLSON, M.R. (1979) *Chem.-Biol. Interact.*, **26**, 57
GARRETT, E.R. and GOTO, S. (1973) *Chem. Pharm. Bull. (Japan)*, **21**, 1811
GINSBERG, A. and GOERDELER, J. (1961) *Chem. Ber.*, **94**, 2043
GOLDWATER, L.J., ROSSO, A.J. and KLEINFELD, M. (1965) *Arch. Environ. Hlth*, **11**, 814
GOODGAME, D.M.L., HAYMAN, P.B. and HATHWAY, D.E. (1982) *Polyhedron*, **1**, 497
GOODGAME, J.I., TROSKO, J.E. and YAGER, J.D. (1976) *Chem.-Biol. Interact.*, **12**, 171
GÖTHE, R., CALLEMAN, C.J., EHRENBERG, L. and WACHTMEISTER, C.A. (1974) *Ambio*, **3**, 234
GOVERNMENT REPORT ANNOUNCEMENTS INDEX (1978) *Bioassay of 1,2-dichloroethane for possible carcinogenicity CAS*, No. 107-06-2. *Gov. Rep. Announc. Index*, **78**(26), 84
GOVERNMENT REPORT ANNOUNCEMENTS INDEX (1979) *Bioassay of 1,2-dibromoethane for possible carcinogenicity*. *Gov. Rep. Announc. Index*, **79**(6), 81
GREEN, T. and HATHWAY, D.E. (1975) *Chem.-Biol. Interact.*, **11**, 545
GREEN, T. and HATHWAY, D.E. (1977) *Chem.-Biol. Interact.*, **17**, 137
GREEN, T. and HATHWAY, D.E. (1978) *Chem.-Biol. Interact.*, **20**, 27
GRICE, H.C., MANNELL, W.A. and ALLMARK, M.G. (1961) *Toxicol. Appl. Pharmacol.*, **3**, 509
GROSS, E. and KOLSCH, F. (1943) *Arch. Gewerbepath. Gewerbehyg.*, **12**, 164
GROSS, H. and FREIBURG, J. (1969) *J. Prakt. Chem.*, **311**, 506
HANSEN, W.H., DAVIS, K.J., FITZHUGH, O.G. and NELSON, A.A. (1963) *Toxicol. Appl. Pharmacol.*, **5**, 105
HARTMAN, C.P., ANDREWS, A.W. and CHUNG, K.-T. (1979) *Infect. Immunol.*, **23**, 686
HARTMAN, C.P., FULK, G.E. and ANDREWS, A.W. (1978) *Mutat. Res.*, **58**, 125
HATHWAY, D.E. (1977) *Environ. Hlth Perspectives*, **21**, 55
HATHWAY, D.E. (ED.) (1979) In *Foreign Compound Metabolism in Mammals*. Vol. 5. pp. 190–243. London: The Chemical Society
HATHWAY, D.E. (1980a) *Chem. Soc. Rev.*, **9**(1), 63
HATHWAY, D.E. (1980b) *Cancer Lett.*, **8**, 263
HATHWAY, D.E. (1984a) *Molecular Aspects of Toxicology*. Chap. 11. London: Royal Society of Chemistry
HATHWAY, D.E. (1984b) *Molecular Aspects of Toxicology*. Chap. 10. London: Royal Society of Chemistry
HATHWAY, D.E. and KOLAR, G.F. (1980) *Chem. Soc. Rev.*, **9**(2), 241
HAWKS, A., FARBER, E. and MAGEE, P.N. (1971/1972) *Chem.-Biol. Interact.*, **4**, 144
HEUBNER, W. (1913) *Naunyn-Schmeidebergs Arch. Pharmakol. Exp. Pathol.*, **72**, 241
HILL, D.L., SHIH, T.-W., JOHNSTON, T.P. and STRUCK, R.F. (1978) *Cancer Res.*, **38**, 2438
HODGSON, E. and CASIDA, J.E. (1962) *J. Agric. Food Chem.*, **10**, 208
HUBERMAN, E., BARTSCH, H. and SACHS, L. (1975) *Int. J. Cancer*, **15**, 539
HUEPER, W.C., WILEY, F.H. and WOLFE, H.D. (1938) *J. Ind. Hyg.*, **20**, 46
HUTSON, D.H., BLAIR, D., HOADLEY, E.C. and PICKERING, B.A. (1971) *Toxicol. Appl. Pharmacol.*, **19**, 378

INTERNATIONAL AGENCY FOR RESEARCH ON CANCER (1975) *IARC Monographs on the Evaluation of Carcinogenic Risk of Chemicals to Man: Aromatic Azo Compounds*, Vol. 8, pp. 41–51, 181–187, 207–215, 257–266. Lyon, France: IARC
IARC (1976) *Monographs on the Evaluation of Carcinogenic Risk of Chemicals to Man: Trichloroethylene*, Vol. 11, pp. 263–276. Lyon, France: IARC
IARC (1979) *Monographs on the Evaluation of Carcinogenic Risk of Chemicals to Man: Dichlorvos*, Vol. 20, pp. 97–127. Lyon, France: IARC
IARC (1982) *Monographs on the Evaluation of Carcinogenic Risk of Chemicals to Man: Industrial Chemicals and Dyestuffs*, Vol. 29, pp. 295–330. Lyon, France: IARC
IRVING, C.C., JANSS, D.H. and RUSSELL, L.T. (1971) *Cancer Res.*, **31**, 387
ITO, N. and FARBER, E. (1966) *J. Natl Cancer Inst.*, **37**, 775
JERINA, D.M. and DALY, J.W. (1977) In *Drug Metabolism from Microbe to Man*. Eds D.V. Parke and R.L. Smith. pp. 13–32. London: Taylor and Francis
JERINA, D.M. and LEHR, R.E. (1977) In *Microsomes and Drug Oxidations: Proceedings of the IIIrd International Symposium*, July 1976. Eds V. Ulbrich, I. Roots, A. Hildebrandt, R.W. Estabrook and A.H. Coney. pp. 709–720. Oxford: Pergamon
JONES, B.K. and HATHWAY, D.E. (1978a) *Br. J. Cancer*, **37**, 411
JONES, B.K. and HATHWAY, D.E. (1978b) *Cancer Lett.*, **5**, 1
KADLUBAR, F.F., MILLER, J.A. and MILLER, E.C. (1977) *Cancer Res.*, **37**, 605
KENSLER, C.J., DEXTER, S.O. and RHOADS, C.P. (1942) *Cancer Res.*, **2**, 1
KIER, L.D., YAMASAKI, E. and AMES, B.N. (1974) *Proc. Natl Acad. Sci. USA*, **71**, 4159
KING, C.M. and PHILLIPS, B. (1968) *Science*, **159**, 1351
KING, C.M., TRAUB, N.R., LOTZ, Z.M. and THISSEN, R.M. (1979) *Cancer Res.*, **39**, 3369
KIRBY, A.H.M. (1947) *Cancer Res.*, **7**, 333
KIRBY, A.H.M. and PEACOCK, P.R. (1947) *J. Pathol. Bacteriol.*, **59**, 1
KÖNIGS, W. and KNORR, E. (1900) *Sitzungsber. Bayr.*, **30**, 103
KOLAR, G.F. (1980) Unpublished results cited in Hathway and Kolar (1980)
KOLAR, G.F. and CARUBELLI, R. (1979) *Cancer Lett.*, **7**, 209
KOLAR, G.F., MAURER, M. and WILDSCHÜTTE, M. (1980) *Cancer Lett.*, **10**, 235
LAM, L.K.T. and WATTENBERG, L.W. (1977) *J. Natl Cancer Inst.*, **58**, 413
LAWLEY, P.D. and THATCHER, C.J. (1970) *Biochem. J.*, **116**, 693
LAZEAR, E.J., SHADDOCK, J.G., BARREN, P.R. and LOUIE, S.C. (1979) *Toxicol. Lett.*, **4**, 519
LE PAGE, R.N. and CHRISTIE, G.S. (1969) *Br. J. Cancer*, **23**, 125
LETTERER, E., NEIDHARDT, K. and KLETT, H. (1944) *Arch. Gewerbepath. Gewerbehyg.*, **12**, 323
LEUENBERGER, S.G. (1912) *Bruns' Beitr. klin. Chir.*, **80**, 208
LHOEST, G., ROBERFROID, M. and MERCIER, M. (1978) *Biomed. Mass Spectrom.*, **5**, 38
LIN, J.-K., JENNAN, K.A., MILLER, J.A. and MILLER, E.C. (1978) *Cancer Res.*, **38**, 2424
LIN, J.-K., MILLER, J.A. and MILLER, E.C. (1977) *Cancer Res.*, **37**, 4430
LLOYD, J.W., MOORE, R.M. and BRESLIN, P. (1975) *J. Occup. Med.*, **17**, 603
LÖFROTH, G. (1978) *Z. Naturforschung*, **33C**, 783
LÖFROTH, G. and AMES, B.N. (1977) *Environmental Mutagen Soc. Abstr.* Annual Meeting, Colorado Springs, Colorado
McCANN, J. and AMES, B.N. (1976) *Ann. N.Y. Acad. Sci.*, **271**, 5
McCANN, J., SIMON, V., STREITWIESER, D. and AMES, B.N. (1975a) *Proc. Natl Acad. Sci. USA*, **73**, 3190
McCANN, J., SPRINGARN, N.E., KOBORI, J. and AMES, B.N. (1975b) *Proc. Natl Acad. Sci. USA*, **72**, 979
MACHLE, W. and GREGORIUS, F. (1948) *Publ. Health Rep., Wash.*, **63**, 114
MAGEE, P.N., MONTESANO, R. and PREUSSMANN, R. (1976) In *Chemical Carcinogens*. Ed. C.E. Searle. A.C.S. Monograph 173, pp. 491–625. Washington, DC: American Chemical Society
MALAVEILLE, C., BARTSCH, H., BARBIN, A., CAMUS, A.M., MONTESANO, R., CROISY, A. et al. (1975) *Biochem. Biophys. Res. Commun.*, **63**, 363
MALLING, H.V. and DE SERRES, H.V. (1969) *Genetics, Princeton*, **61**, 39
MALTONI, C. (1976a) *Ann. N.Y. Acad. Sci.*, **271**, 431
MALTONI, C. (1976b) *Ann. N.Y. Acad. Sci.*, **271**, 444
MALTONI, C. (1976c) In *Environmental Pollution and Carcinogenic Risks*. Eds C. Rosenfeld and W. Davis. Institut National de la Santé et de la Recherche Médicale, Symposia Series. Vol. 52, pp. 127–149 (International Agency for Research on Cancer, Scientific Publications, vol. 13). Paris: Inserm
MALTONI, C. (1977a) In *Origins of Human Cancer*. Eds H.H. Hiatt, J.D. Watson and J.A. Winsten. Proc. Cold Spring Harbor Lab., Cold Spring Harbor, Massachusetts
MALTONI, C. (1977b) *Adv. Tumor Prev. Detect. Charact.*, **3**, 216
MALTONI, C. and LEFEMINE, G. (1974a) *Atti Accad. naz. Lincei, Cl. Sci. Fis. Mat. Nat. Rend.*, [8] **56**, 1

MALTONI, C. and LEFEMINE, G. (1974b) *Environ. Res.*, **7**, 387
MALTONI, C. and LEFEMINE, G. (1975) *Ann. N.Y. Acad. Sci.*, **246**, 195
MANCUSO, T.F. and HUEPER, W.C. (1951) *Ind. Med. Surg.*, **20**, 358
MANCUSO, T.F. and EL-ATTAR, A.A. (1967) *J. Occup. Med.*, **9**, 277
MANNELL, W.A. (1964) *Food Cosmet. Toxicol.*, **2**, 169
MARSHALL, A.H.E. (1953) *Acta Pathol. Microbiol. Scand.*, **33**, 1
MILLER, J.A. (1970) *Cancer Res.*, **30**, 559
MILLER, J.A., CRAMER, J.W. and MILLER, E.C. (1960) *Cancer Res.*, **20**, 950
MILLER, J.A. and MILLER, E.C. (1971) *J. Natl Cancer Inst.*, **47**, v
MONTESANO, R. and BARTSCH, H. (1978) *Mutat. Res.*, **32**, 179
MORGAN, J.G. (1958) *Br. J. Ind. Med.*, **15**, 224
MORTON, K.C., KING, C.M. and BAETCKE, K.P. (1979) *Cancer Res.*, **39**, 3107
MOSS, R.A. (1974) *Acc. Chem. Res.*, **7**, 421
MÜLLER, E. and HAISS, H. (1962) *Chem. Ber.*, **95**, 1255
NAGATA, Y. and MATSUMOTO, H. (1969) *Proc. Soc. Exp. Biol. Med.*, **132**, 383
NELSON, A.A. and WOODARD, G. (1953) *J. Natl Cancer Inst.*, **13**, 1497
NISHIOKA, H. (1975a) *Mutat. Res.*, **31**, 185
NISHIOKA, H. (1975b) *Jap. J. Genet.*, **50**, 485
NONY, C.R., BOWMAN, M.C., CAIRNS, T., LOWRY, L.K. and TOLOS, W.P. (1980) *J. Analyt. Toxicol.*, **4**, 132
ODASHIMA, S. and HASHIMOTO, Y. (1968) *Gann*, **59**, 131
OESCH, F., SCHMASSMANN, H. and BENTLEY, P. (1978) *Biochem. Pharmacol.*, **27**, 17
OKA, K., MATSUYAMA, K., ARAKI, Y. and OONEDA, G. (1957) *Gann*, **48**, 573
OLSON, W.A., HABERMANN, R.T., WEISBURGER, E.K., WARD, J.M. and WEISBURGER, J.H. (1973) *J. Natl Cancer Inst.*, **51**, 1973
OONEDA, G., MATSUYAMA, K., OKA, K., NINOMIYA, S., ARAKI, Y. and TAKANO, M. (1957) *Gunma J. Med. Sci.*, **6**, 295
OSTERMAN-GOLKAR, S. (1974) *Mutat. Res.*, **24**, 219
OTTENWAELDER, H., LAIB, R.J. and BOLT, H.M. (1979) *Arch. Toxicol.*, **41**, 290
PAPACHARALAMPOUS, N.X. (1966) *Frank. Z. Pathol.*, **75**, 74
PARK, K.K., ARCHER, M.C. and WISHNOK, J.S. (1980) *Chem.-Biol. Interact.*, **29**, 139
PETRILLI, F.L. and DE FLORA, S. (1977) *Appl. Environ. Microbiol.*, **33**, 805
PHILLIPS, D.H. and SIMS, P. (1979) In *Chemical Carcinogens and DNA*. Ed. P.L. Grover. Vol. 2, pp. 29–58. Boca Raton, Florida: CRC Press
PLISS, G.B. (1965) *Gig. Tr. prof. Zabol.*, **9**, 18
PLISS, G.B. and ZABEZHINSKY, M.A. (1970) *J. Natl Cancer Inst.*, **45**, 283
POIRIER, L.A., MILLER, J.A., MILLER, E.C. and SATO, K. (1967) *Cancer Res.*, **27**, 1600
POTT, P. (1775) *Chirurgical Works*. London: Hower, Clarke and Pollins
PREUSSMANN, R., DRUCKREY, H., IVANKOVIC, S. and VON HODENBERG, A. (1969) *Ann. N.Y. Acad. Sci.*, **163**, 697
PROUGH, R.A. (1973) *Arch. Biochem. Biophys.*, **158**, 442
RADOMSKI, J.L. and BRILL, E. (1970) *Science*, **167**, 992
RADOMSKI, J.L. and BRILL, E. (1971) *Arch. Toxicol.*, **28**, 159
RADOMSKI, J.L., BRILL, E., DEICHMAN, W.B. and GLASS, E.M. (1971) *Cancer Res.*, **31**, 1461
RADOMSKI, J.L., HEARN, W.L., RADOMSKI, T., MORENO, H. and SCOTT, W.E. (1977) *Cancer Res.*, **37**, 1757
RANNUG, U. and BËYE, B. (1979) *Chem.-Biol. Interact.*, **24**, 265
RANNUG, U., GÖTHE, R. and WACHTMEISTER, C.A. (1976) *Chem.-Biol. Interact.*, **12**, 251
RANNUG, U., JOHANSSON, A., RAMEL, C. and WACHTMEISTER, C.A. (1974) *Ambio*, **3**, 194
ROBINSON, R. (1946) *Br. Med. J.*, **i**, 945
ROE, F.J.C. (1978) *Ann. Occup. Hyg.*, **21**, 323
ROE, F.J.C., GRANT, G.A. and MILLICAN, D.M. (1967) *Nature*, **216**, 375
SALMON, A.G. (1976) *Cancer Lett.*, **2**, 109
SASAKI, T. and YOSHIDA, T. (1935) *Virchows Arch. Pathol. Anat. Physiol.*, **295**, 175
SCOTT, T.S. (1952) *Br. J. Ind. Med.*, **9**, 127
SHANK, R.C. and MAGEE, P.N. (1967) *Biochem. J.*, **105**, 521
SHUBIK, P. and CLAYSON, D.B. (1976) In *Environmental Pollution and Carcinogenic Risks*. Eds C. Rosenfeld and W. Davis. Institut National de la Santé et de la recherche Médicale, Symposia Series, Vol. 52, pp. 241–252 (International Agency for Research on Cancer, Scientific Publications, vol. 13). Paris: Inserm
SIMPSON, C.L. (1952) *Br. J. Exp. Pathol.*, **33**, 524
SIMS, P. and GROVER, P.L. (1974) *Adv. Cancer Res.*, **20**, 165
SINGH, A.R., LAWRENCE, W.H. and AUTIAN, J. (1972) *J. Dent. Res.*, **51**, 1632

SLAGA, T.J. and BRACKEN, W.R. (1977) *Cancer Res.,* **37**, 1631
SLAGA, T.J., BRACKEN, W.R., GLEASON, G., LEVIN, W., YAGI, H., JERINA, D.M. et al. (1979) *Cancer Res.,* **39**, 67
SPANNAGEL, H. (1953) *Arbeitsmed.,* **28**, 92
STILLWELL, W.G., CARMAN, M.J., BELL, L. and HORNING, M.G. (1974) *Drug. Metabol. Disposition,* **2**, 489
STOUT, D.L. and BECKER, F.F. (1979) *Cancer Res.,* **39**, 1168
SUNDERMAN, F.W. (1968) *Dis. Chest.,* **54**, 41
TANAKA, K.-I. (1980) *Jap. J. Ind. Hlth,* **22**, 194
TOTH, B. (1972) *Proc. Am. Assoc. Cancer Res.,* **13**, 34
TOTH, B. (1973) *J. Natl Cancer Inst.,* **50**, 181
TSUTSUI, H. (1918) *Gann,* **12**, 17
ÜBELIN, F. VON and PLETSCHER, A. (1954) *Schweiz. med. Wochenschr.,* **84**, 917
VAN DUUREN, B.L. (1975) *Ann. N.Y. Acad. Sci.,* **246**, 258
VELEMINSKY, J., OSTERMAN-GOLKAR, S. and EHRENBERG, L. (1970) *Mutat. Res.,* **10**, 169
VENITT, S. (1974) *Nature,* **250**, 493
VIOLA, P.L., BIGOTTI, A. and CAPUTO, A. (1971) *Cancer Res.,* **31**, 516
WATTENBERG, L.W. (1978) *Adv. Cancer Res.,* **26**, 197
WEISBURGER, E.K., EVARTS, R.P. and WENK, M.L. (1977) *Food Cosmet. Toxicol.,* **15**, 139
WEISBURGER, J.H., YAMAMOTO, R.S., WILLIAMS, G.M., GRANTHAM, P.H., MATSUSHIMA, T. and WEISBURGER, E.K. (1972) *Cancer Res.,* **32**, 491
WIEBECKE, B., LÖHRS, U., GIMMY, J. and EDER, M. (1969) *Z. Ges. Exp. Med.,* **149**, 277
WILLIAMS, M.H.C. (1962) *Acta Unio Int. Contra Cancrum,* **18**, 676
WILLIAMS, W.J. (1958) *Br. J. Ind. Med.,* **15**, 235
WILLSTÄTTER, R. and KUBLI, H. (1908) *Ber. dtsch chem. Ges.,* **41**, 1936
WISLOCKI, P.G., BORCHERT, P., MILLER, J.A. and MILLER, E.C. (1976) *Cancer Res.,* **36**, 1686
YAGI, H., THAKKER, D.R., HERNANDEZ, O., KOREEDA, M. and JERINA, D.M. (1977) *J. Am. Chem. Soc.,* **99**, 1604
YAMIGAWA, K. and ICHIKAWA, K. (1915) *Mitt. med. fak. Jap. Univ. (Kaiserl),* **15**, 295
YAMAMOTO, R.S., GLASS, R.M., FRANKEL, H.H., WEISBURGER, E.K. and WEISBURGER, J.H. (1968) *Toxicol. Appl. Pharmacol.,* **13**, 108
YANG, S.K. and GELBOIN, H.V. (1976) *Biochem. Pharmacol.,* **25**, 2221
YOSHIDA, T. (1932) *Proc. Imp. Acad, Japan,* **8**, 464
YOSHIDA, T. (1933) *Trans. Jap. Pathol. Soc.,* **23**, 636

Chapter 3
Authenticated interactions with nucleic acid

The aphorism 'Ogni cosa ha cagione (nothing happens without a cause)' manifestly applies to neoplastic change, and amongst other experiments, those of Berward and Sachs (1965) prove that normal cells are transformed into tumour cells by chemical carcinogens. Host factors undoubtedly contribute to the predisposition of a living mammal to cancer and, in some cases, the cells of healthy, unexposed individuals seem to have already undergone some changes in that direction (Miller and Todaro, 1969; Kopelovich, Conlon and Pollack, 1977). Nevertheless, the transfer of a permanent heritable change in properties through successive generations of cells is absolutely essential to the transformation of normal cells into tumour cells. This condition is fulfilled through the exposure to a chemical carcinogen and by the resulting chemical modification of genetic material that induces somatic mutation. Thus, nucleic acids act as receptors for the reactive intermediates initiating the cancer process.

The present chapter describes the interaction of reactive carcinogen intermediates (Chapter 2) with DNA and takes account of the possibility that chemical changes to some RNA macromolecules, which may act as templates for DNA synthesis, might modify DNA indirectly in a significant way.

Aromatic amines and amino-azo dyes

The gentle chemical reaction (S_N1) between deoxyguanine (1) (*Scheme 3.1*) and N-sulphonoxy-N-(2-fluorenyl)acetamide (2), the generally accepted ultimate carcinogen (Chapter 2) of N-(2-fluorenyl)acetamide (2AAF), afforded a major product N-[(deoxyguanosin-8-yl)-2-fluorenyl]acetamide (3) and a minor product N-[(3-deoxyguanosin-N^2-yl)-2-fluorenyl]acetamide (4), which were identical in every respect with the products obtained from hydrolysates of the modified DNA, extracted from the liver of rats, injected with N-hydroxy-N-(2-fluorenyl)acetamide (Westra, Kriek and Hittenhausen, 1976). In earlier work (Kriek *et al.*, 1967; Miller and Miller, 1971), the nucleoside analogue (3) had been identified as a reaction product.

In other experiments, the modified DNA obtained by reaction of either 4-acetamido-4'-fluorobiphenyl or 4-amino-4'-fluorobiphenyl with rat-liver and

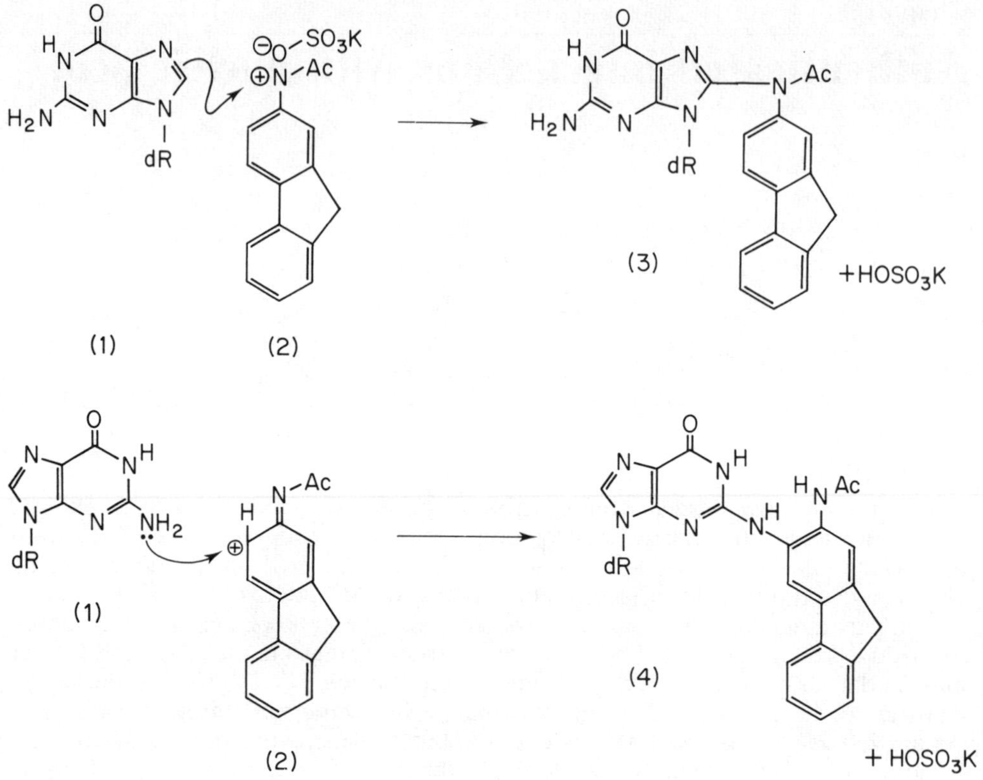

Scheme 3.1

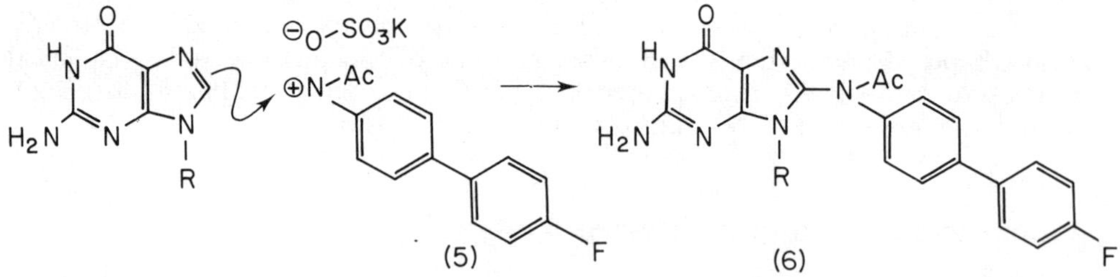

Scheme 3.2

rat-kidney DNA gave, on hydrolysis, either N-(deoxyguanosin-8-yl)-4-acetamido-4'-fluorobiphenyl (6) (*Scheme 3.2*) or N-(deoxyguanosin-8-yl)-4-amino-4'-fluorobiphenyl (Kriek and Hengeveld, 1978). The synthetic N-KOSO$_3$-4-acetamido-4'-fluorobiphenyl (5) was found to be twice as reactive as 4-acetamido-4'-fluorobiphenyl towards the deoxyguanosine residues of DNA (Kriek and Hengeveld, 1978).

Deoxyguanosin-8-yl analogues (q.v.) came to be regarded as the prototype 'adducts' of aromatic amine carcinogens, formed in the liver DNA, but this concept loses caste somewhat with the finding (Kriek, 1972) that, for example, (3) rather than (4) was eliminated preferentially from the modified DNA. The argument has been advanced, however, that such DNA repair may contribute *per se* to 2AAF carcinogenicity, but this is not very convincing. In fact, further chemical investigations revealed that other *N*-acetoxy-*N*-arylacetamides, *N*-acetoxy-2-acetamidophenanthrene (Scribner and Naimy, 1973; 1975) and *N*-acetoxy-4-aminostilbene (Miller and Miller, 1969), attacked the adenine as well as the guanine bases in DNA. It may be relevant also that the mutagenicity of *N*-acetoxy-*N*-(2-fluorenyl)acetamide in bacteriophage has been attributed in large

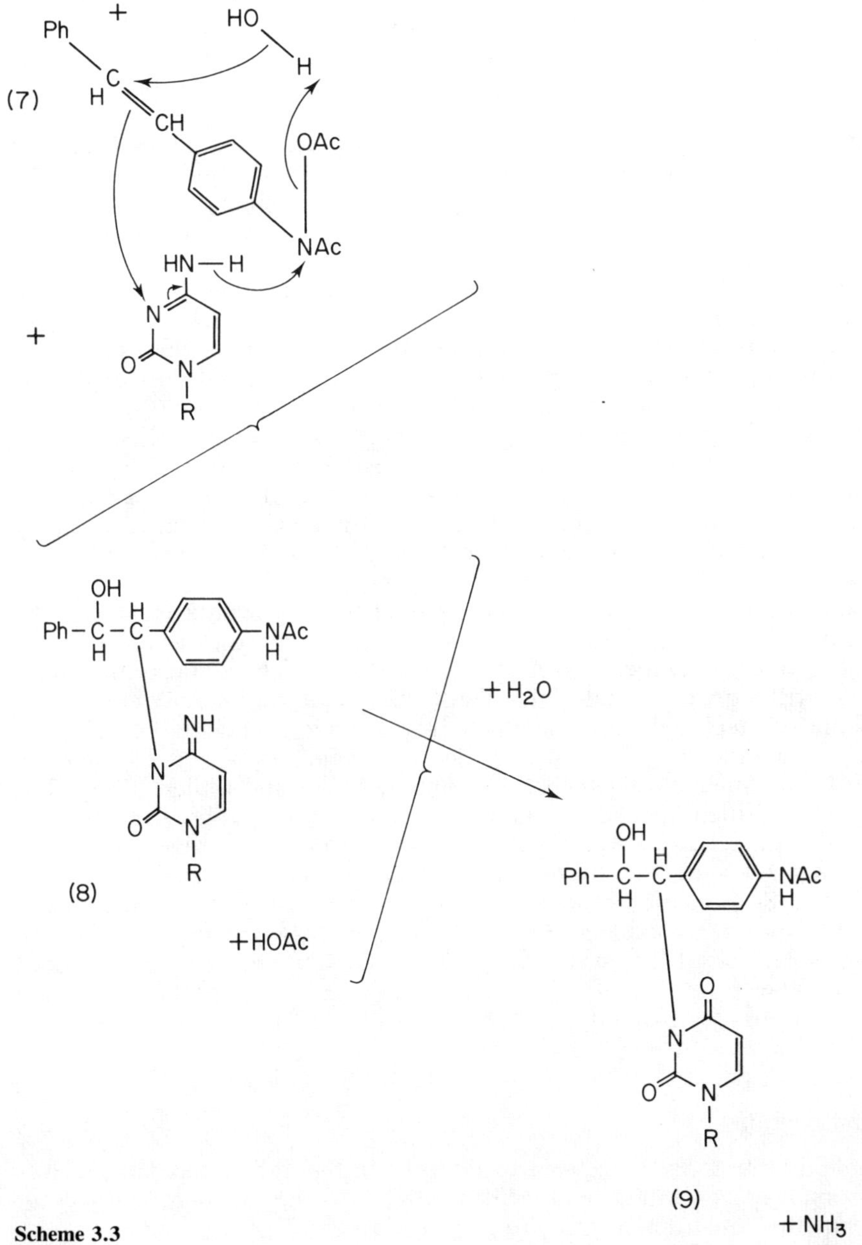

Scheme 3.3

50 Authenticated interactions with nucleic acid

degree to damage at an adenine–thymine locus (Corbett, Heidelberger and Dove, 1970).

Detailed examination (Scribner and Scribner, 1979; Scribner *et al.*, 1979) of the chemical reactions between *N*-acetoxy-4-acetamidostilbene (7) and cytidine, adenosine and guanosine, as well as of (7) with homopolynucleotides and RNA *in vitro* showed many nucleoside analogues to be formed. The fact that compound (7) attacks many sites in both RNA and DNA strongly suggests that it behaves more like a classical alkylating agent than the previously reported *N*-acetoxy-*N*-arylacetamides did (*see above*). The target organs for *N*-acetamidostilbene are, however, the same as those for the other *N*-arylacetamides. The major product from the reaction of (7) with cytidine is a deamination product, 1-(4-acetamidophenyl)-1-(3-uridyl)-2-hydroxy-2-phenylethane (9) (*Scheme 3.3*). A cyclic mechanism is tentatively proposed by the present writer, whereby (7) reacts with cytidine and one molecule of water with alkylation at N-1, and elimination of the elements of acetic acid, to give a hypothetical intermediate (8). Whence, hydrolysis of the imino group in the 6-position affords (9). Similar alkylation at N-6 of adenosine with elimination of the elements of acetic acid leads to formation of 1-(4-acetamidophenyl)-1-(N^6-adenosyl)-2-hydroxy-2-phenylethane (10) (*Scheme 3.4*), and at N-1 of adenosine with elimination of the elements of acetic acid leads to formation of (11), which by cyclization through the elimination of the elements of water affords the imidazopurine derivative, 3-(β-D-ribosyl)-7-phenyl-8-(4-acetamidophenyl)-7,8-dihydro-imidazo[2,1-*i*]purine (12) (*Scheme 3.5*). Similar alkylation at N-1 of guanosine with elimination of the elements of acetic acid affords the major adduct, 1-(4-acetamidophenyl)-1-(1-guanosyl)-2-hydroxy-2-phenylethane (13) (*Scheme 3.6*). A minor adduct appears also to be a 1-guanosyl derivative, whereas two other minor adducts are O^6-guanosyl derivatives, as they gave 1-(4-acetamidophenyl)-2-phenylethane-1,2-diol by acid hydrolysis (Scribner *et al.*, 1979).

Whilst none of the foregoing substances has ever been a bulk chemical, the examples which have been cited would appear to shed light on the reactivity of commercial aromatic amines, such as 1- and 2-naphthylamines and their derivatives, with genetic material. Thus, the reactive metabolite of 1-naphthylamine, 1-naphthylhydroxylamine (14) (*Scheme 3.7*) with DNA under slightly acidic conditions (pH 5) gives nucleoside analogues with 3–20 naphthyl residues/1000 monomer units in DNA (Kadlubar, Miller and Miller, 1978). The major adduct was identified as *N*-(deoxyguanosin-O^6-yl)-1-naphthylamine (15), and two other adducts as 2-(deoxyguanosin-O^6-yl)-1-naphthylamine (16) and a decomposition product of (16). Arylnitrenium and arylcarbenium ion participation, and in fact the S_N1 reaction mechanism postulated (*Scheme 3.7*), were neatly established by means of stable isotopes: the former through isotope exchange following the solvolysis of (14) in acidic $H_2^{18}O$, and the latter through simultaneous formation of the products of hydration, viz. 1-amino-2-naphthol (17) and 4-amino-1-naphthol (18) (Kadlubar, Miller and Miller, 1978).

Proteins and peptides

Considerable attention has been paid to the protein binding of carcinogens ever since the first report (Miller and Miller, 1947) of the covalent binding of 4-dimethylamino-azobenzene (DAB) to rat-liver protein.

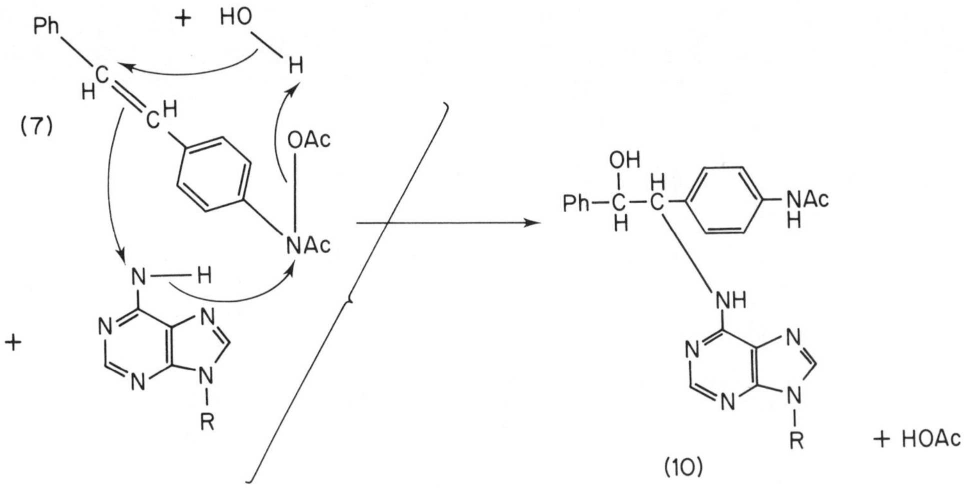

Scheme 3.4

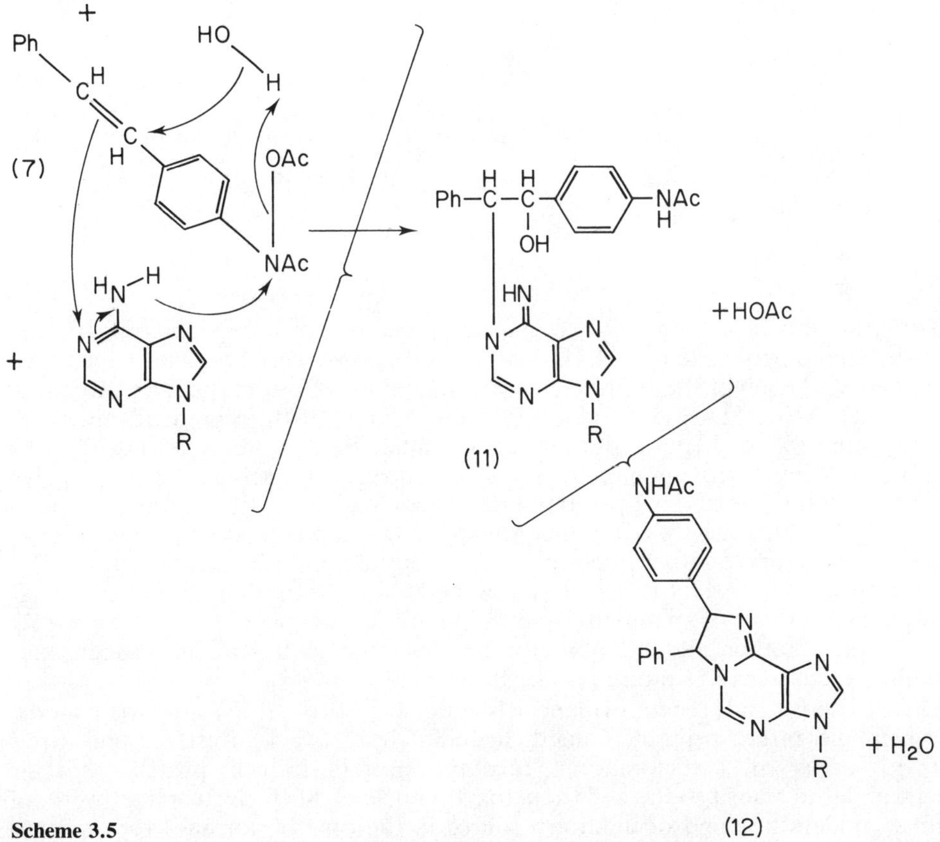

Scheme 3.5

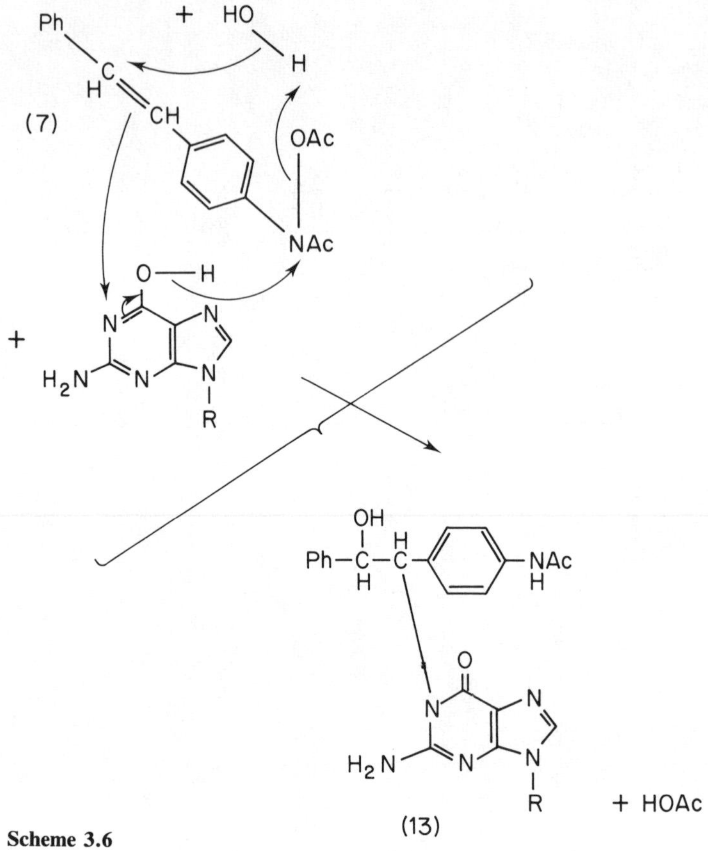

52 Authenticated interactions with nucleic acid

Scheme 3.6

The structures of the polar dyes (Chapter 2) resulting from reaction of DAB and 4-methylamino-azobenzene (MAB) with methionine and tyrosine have been identified, and each of these products was isolated as well from the liver protein of rats dosed DAB or MAB (De Baun, Miller and Miller, 1970). A great advance with regard to the role of hepatic glutathione was made by Ketterer et al. (1979), who found that N-benzoyloxy-4-methylamino-azobenzene, an analogue of the reactive DAB metabolite, reacted with glutathione *in vitro* to give a major product (19; R = R^2 = H; R^1 = SG) (where SG = glutathion-S-yl), a minor product (19; R = R^1 = H; R^2 = 2-SG), and another minor product, identified provisionally as (19; R = R^1 = H; R^2 = 4-SG). Analysis of the biliary metabolites from rats dosed with DAB showed the presence of an amino-azo dye–glutathione adduct (19; R = R^2 = H; R^1 = SG) and another adduct, partially characterized as a 4-amino-azobenzene-glutathione derivative (Ketterer et al., 1979).

On the other hand, recent evidence (Mainigi and Sorof, 1977) supports a model in which the target protein, named 'ligandin' by Litwack, Ketterer and Arias (1971), serves as a cytoplasmic receptor protein, which protects specific electrophiles in transit to the cell (hepatocyte) nucleus. Such electrophiles were, of course, unidentified and of unknown source in the case of normal liver, and are

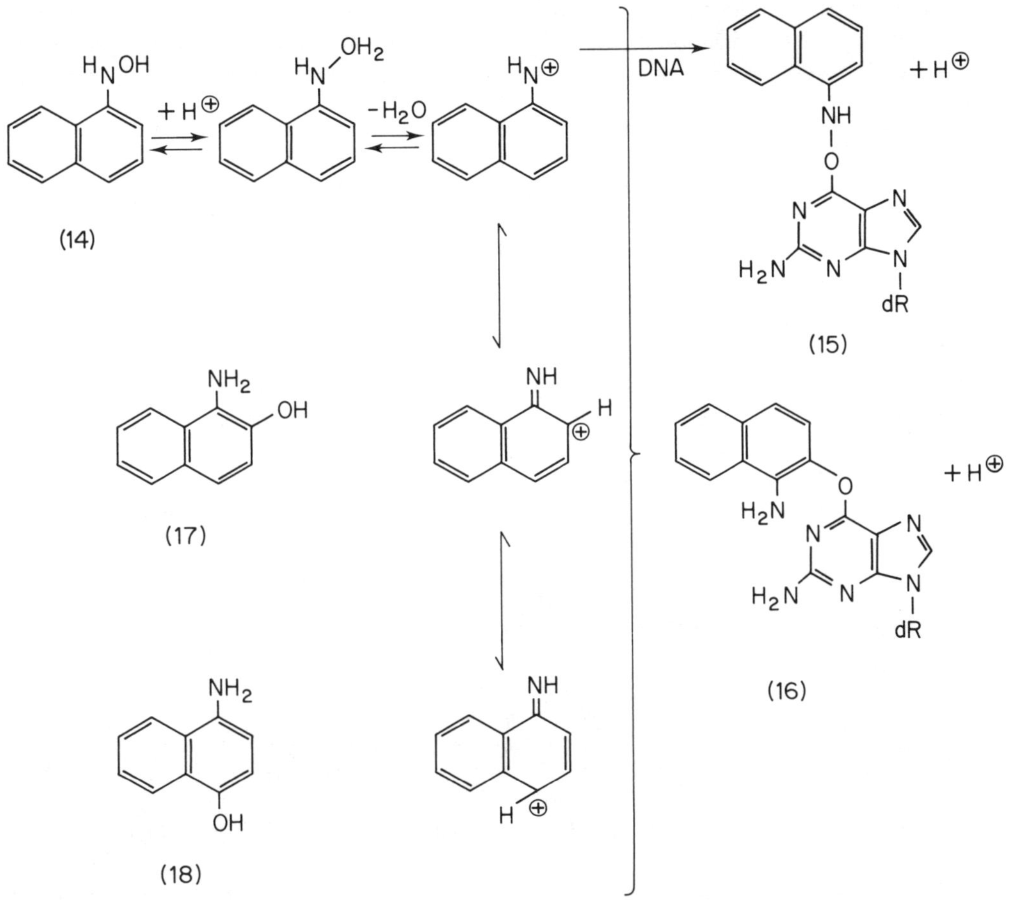

Aromatic amines and amino-azo dyes 53

Scheme 3.7

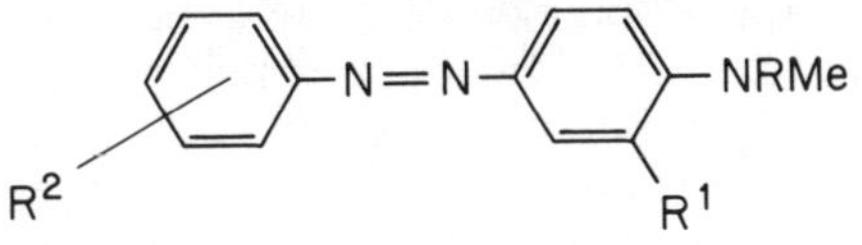

(19)

reactive carcinogen metabolites (Chapter 2) in the case of the liver during chemical carcinogenesis as, for example, incurred by amino-azo dyes. This model agrees largely with other concurrent work (Litwack, Ketterer and Arias, 1971; Ketterer *et al.*, 1975). The cytosolic protein (and rat ligandin has been identified as glutathione S-transferase-1,1) is the main reagent, for example, for reactive azocarcinogen metabolite throughout hepatocarcinogenesis. The interaction in question is specific to the protein (Sorof *et al.*, 1963, 1970; Sorof and Young, 1973), to the carcinogen (Sorof *et al.*, 1970), and to the organ (Sani *et al.*, 1972). Ultimate azocarcinogen metabolite appears to react non-covalently with target protein (Litwack, Ketterer and Arias, 1971; Mainigi and Sorof, 1977), which undergoes reversible conformational change to a more compact configuration. Such a complex might be supposed to provide the reactive azocarcinogen metabolite with a protective hydrophobic environment during its transport to the nuclei and, in fact, a low concentration of the complex has been detected in liver-cell nuclei (Bakay and Sorof, 1964; Bakay, Sorof and Siebert, 1969). The conformationally altered protein specifically directs covalent reaction between the ultimate azocarcinogen metabolite and (nuclear) DNA.

RNA

As far as the present writer is aware, there is no case where the mammalian carcinogenicity of an aromatic amine, which does not react with DNA, can be attributed to its covalent reaction with RNA. The greater binding of some aromatic amine carcinogens to tRNA in comparison with that to rRNA may mirror only the fact that, in the cytoplasm, tRNA is more exposed than rRNA is to chemical attack (Kriek, 1974).

Nitrosamines and 3-alkyl-1-phenyltriazenes

The Me-N_2^+ ions generating *N*-methyl-*N*-nitrosourea (MNU) and *N*-methyl-*N'*-nitro-*N*-nitrosoguanidine (MNNG) (Chapter 2) give high yields of O-alkylation products; the ratio of O^6-methylguanine to 7-methylguanine being about 0.11 (and the proportion of phosphotriesters being about 0.2) (Frei and Lawley, 1976; Swenson, Farmer and Lawley, 1976). In the case of the Me-N_2^+ generating 3-methyl-1-phenyltriazene (Chapter 2), the ratio of O^6-methylguanine to 7-methylguanine ranges from 0.08 for liver DNA through 0.12 for DNA from the kidneys and lungs to 0.15 for that from the brain, which is one of the principal target organs for tumours (Bartsch *et al.*, 1977). In addition, reaction of MNU or MNNG with DNA gives a number of minor products, including 1- and 3-methyladenine (so that the ratio of 3-methyladenine to 7-methylguanine is about 0.13), 3-methylpyrimidines and a somewhat larger proportion of 7-methyladenine and 3-methylguanine (Lawley, 1974, 1976; Pegg, 1977). In this connection, the reaction of MPT with DNA *in vivo* also gave 3-methyladenine and 3-methylpyrimidines (Marginson, Likhachev and Kolar, 1979). The indirectly acting *N,N*-dimethylnitrosamine (DMN) is also Me-N_2^+ generating (Chapter 2), and the pattern of DNA methylation products derived from DMN *in vivo* (Craddick, 1973; O'Connor, Capps and Craig, 1973; Nicoll, Swann and Pegg, 1977) follows essentially that yielded by chemically activated MNU (*see above*), and thereby reflects the common methylation mechanisms via Me-N_2^+ ions (*Scheme 3.8*), which are more correctly described as S_N2 than S_N1. In addition, the relative amounts of methylated bases produced by the indirectly acting 3,3-dimethyl-1-phenyltriazene (DMPT) (Kleihues, Kolar and Marginson, 1976) were essentially similar to the ones given by MPT (Marginson, Likhachev and Kolar, 1979), and again inferring that both DMPT and MPT react with DNA through Me-N_2^+ ions (Chapter 2).

In the case of ethylation, nucleic acid is alkylated to a lesser extent than by methylation, and the phosphotriesters may comprise up to 70 per cent of the

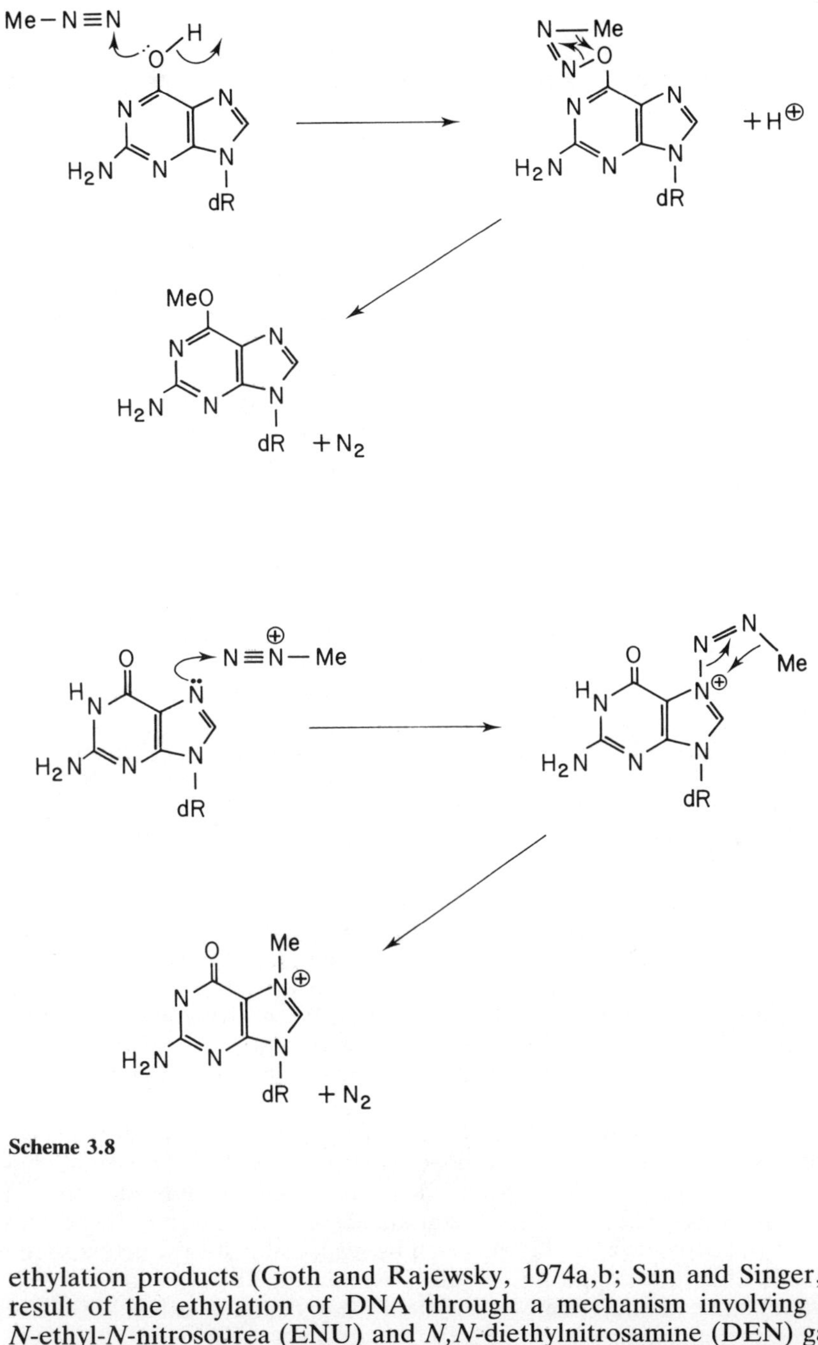

Scheme 3.8

ethylation products (Goth and Rajewsky, 1974a,b; Sun and Singer, 1975). As a result of the ethylation of DNA through a mechanism involving Et-N$_2^+$ ions, *N*-ethyl-*N*-nitrosourea (ENU) and *N,N*-diethylnitrosamine (DEN) gave a ratio of O^6-ethylguanine to 7-ethylguanine ranging from 0.48 to at least 0.70 (Sun and Singer, 1975). 3-Ethyladenine is the third most abundant product, after O^6-ethylguanine and 7-ethylguanine, in DNA ethylation (Goth and Rajewsky, 1974a,b; Sun and Singer, 1975).

Metals

cis-Diaminedichloroplatinum (II) is a mutagen under standard test conditions (Beck and Brubaker, 1975; Monti-Bragadini, Tanaro and Banfi, 1975; Lecointe *et al.*, 1977), and it is the parent compound of a series of antineoplastic agents (Roberts and Thomson, 1979), whereas the *trans*-isomers are inactive. Pt(en)Cl$_2$ reacts with nucleosides in the order guanosine > adenosine ≃ deoxycytidine (Robins, 1973). It is apparent (Singer, 1975) that these platinum S$_N$2 electrophiles show approximately the same specificity (Goodgame *et al.*, 1975; Mansy *et al.*, 1978) towards DNA nucleophilic sites, i.e. guanine > adenine > cytosine, as diethyl sulphate (DES), dimethyl sulphate (DMS) and methyl methanesulphonate (MMS). Under neutral conditions, these reagents alkylate preferentially N-7 of guanine, N-1 of adenine and N-3 of cytosine, and the degree of selectivity shown is consistent with a mechanism of interaction with DNA involving the bimolecular displacement of chlorine. There is no crystallographic evidence for bidentate binding of these Pt electrophiles to guanine residues of DNA (Goodgame *et al.*, 1975; cf. Roberts and Thomson, 1979).

Vinyl chloride

Green and Hathway (1978) established, by the mass fragmentograms which they published, the presence of the imidazo cyclization products of deoxyadenosine (dA) and deoxycytidine (dC), viz. 9-(β-D-2'-deoxyribofuranosyl)imidazo[2,1-*i*]purine (etheno-dA) (20) (*Scheme 3.9*) and 9-(β-D-2'-deoxyribofuranosyl)imidazo[1,2-*c*]pyrimid-2[1*H*]-one (etheno-dC) (21) in chromatographic fractions of the enzyme hydrolysates resulting from the modified hepatic DNA of surviving rats, which had been exposed long-term to vinyl chloride in their drinking water (250 ppm) (*see also* Hathway, 1977). A high incidence of these rats died with liver haemangiosarcoma, out of the large group which had been exposed in this way to vinyl chloride during a 2-year experiment (IARC, 1979). Green and Hathway (1978) implicitly inferred that their results belonged to the causal mechanism, i.e. that formation of (20) and (21) might represent promutagenic lesions in the extrahepatocellular liver-tissue DNA of animals exposed to vinyl chloride. In addition, the formation of (20) and (21) *in vivo* and in model experiments, in which vinyl chloride-derived chloroethylene oxide or its chloroacetaldehyde rearrangement product had reacted with calf-thymus DNA, implied a common mechanism.

There is a strong supposition (Oesch and Doerjer, 1982) that the acid hydrolysate of DNA, which had been modified by reaction with chloroacetaldehyde under different reaction conditions from those employed in the preparation of poly(dC–dG) templates (Hall *et al.*, 1981), contained some etheno-dG (22) besides a preponderance of (20) and (21); (22) may well be responsible for the errors found (Hall *et al.*, 1981; Chapter 4) opposite guanine bases during nucleic acid synthesis. Hall *et al.* (1981) had been uncertain whether such a supposition was tenable as, for example, N^2,3-ethenoguanine was synthesized (Sattsangi, Leonard and Frihart, 1977) under different conditions from those used in related work (Barrio, Secrist and Leonard, 1972; Green and Hathway, 1978). Although compound (22) has not yet been isolated from the liver DNA of rats subjected to long-term exposure to vinyl chloride, it is reasonable to consider that etheno-dA (20), etheno-dC (21) and

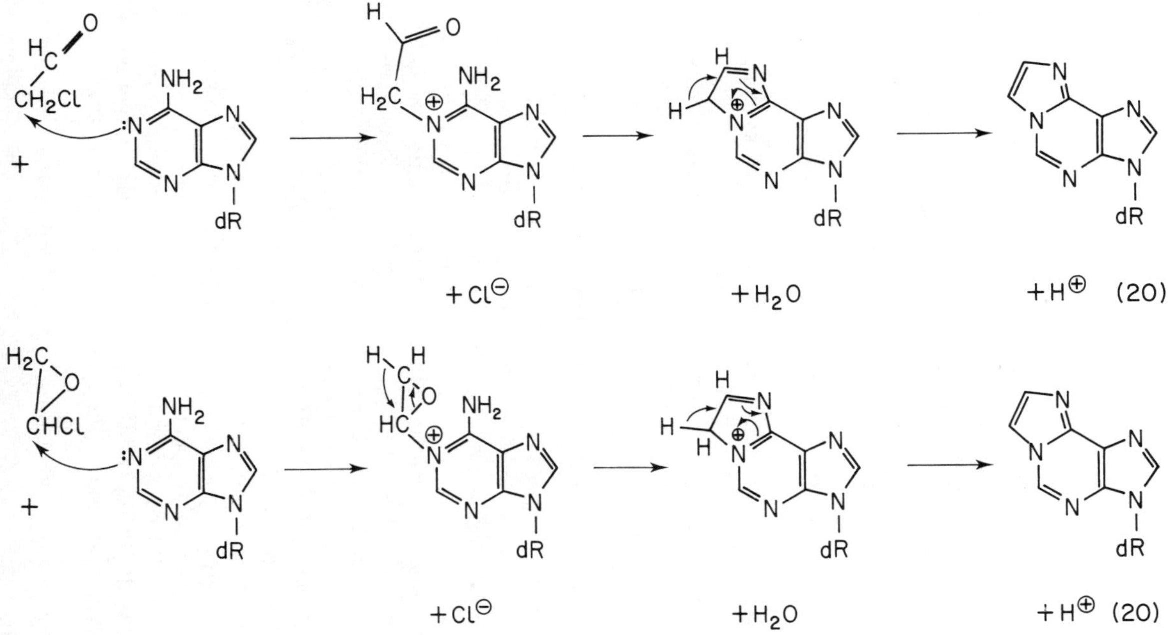

Scheme 3.9

58 Authenticated interactions with nucleic acid

(20)   (21)   (22)

etheno-dG (22) contribute to the causal mechanism of vinyl chloride carcinogenicity.

In this case (*Scheme 3.9*), initial S$_N$2 alkylation occurred at the most nucleophilic ring-nitrogen (N-1 of the dA residues and N-3 of the dC and dG residues), and was followed successively by loss of the elements of water with ring closure between the oxo group and the amino group belonging to C-6 of the dA residues (to C-4 of the dC residues and to C-2 of the dG residues), and by proton loss (Hathway, 1980; Hathway and Kolar, 1980).

Laib and Bolt (1977, 1978) reported chromatographic evidence for the presence of the corresponding ribonucleoside analogues, etheno-A and etheno-C, in fractions of the enzyme hydrolysate of the liver RNA of rats, which had been exposed to a massive acute dose of [^{14}C]vinyl chloride, and they confirmed their results with incubations of rat-liver microsomes, [^{14}C]vinyl chloride and the appropriate polynucleotide, fortified with NADPH.

Consideration of molecular models shows that:

(a) The imidazole ring in vinyl chloride nucleoside analogues is coplanar with the rest of the molecule, and this observation finds support in X-ray crystallography (Wang et al., 1974; Wang, Barrio and Paul, 1976).
(b) The imidazole ring in these nucleoside analogues shields 2 normal hydrogen-bonding positions (Hathway and Kolar, 1980).
(c) In the case of etheno-dC (or etheno-C), the second ring confers on the cytosine residue the dimensions of adenine, with the result that etheno-dC would be expected to simulate dA nucleosides/nucleotides in replication (Barbin et al., 1981; Hall et al., 1981) and etheno-C the A residues in transcription (Spengler and Singer, 1981).
(d) The misincorporation envisaged in these biological processes would be facilitated by complex formation involving base-pairing (Chapter 4) of protonated molecular species, which were invoked (Topal and Fresco, 1976) to extend the Watson–Crick concept for complementary base-pairing.
(e) The relatively bulky imidazole ring resembles an alkyl substituent and effectively blocks one of the available base-pairing sites.

Glycidaldehyde

The imidazo cyclization of purine and pyrimidine residues in DNA that has been established for vinyl chloride *in vivo* (Green and Hathway, 1978) (*Scheme 3.9*) appears to be an important biochemical lesion (Scribner et al., 1979) (*Scheme 3.5*). In another example, glycidaldehyde which contains both an aldehyde and an

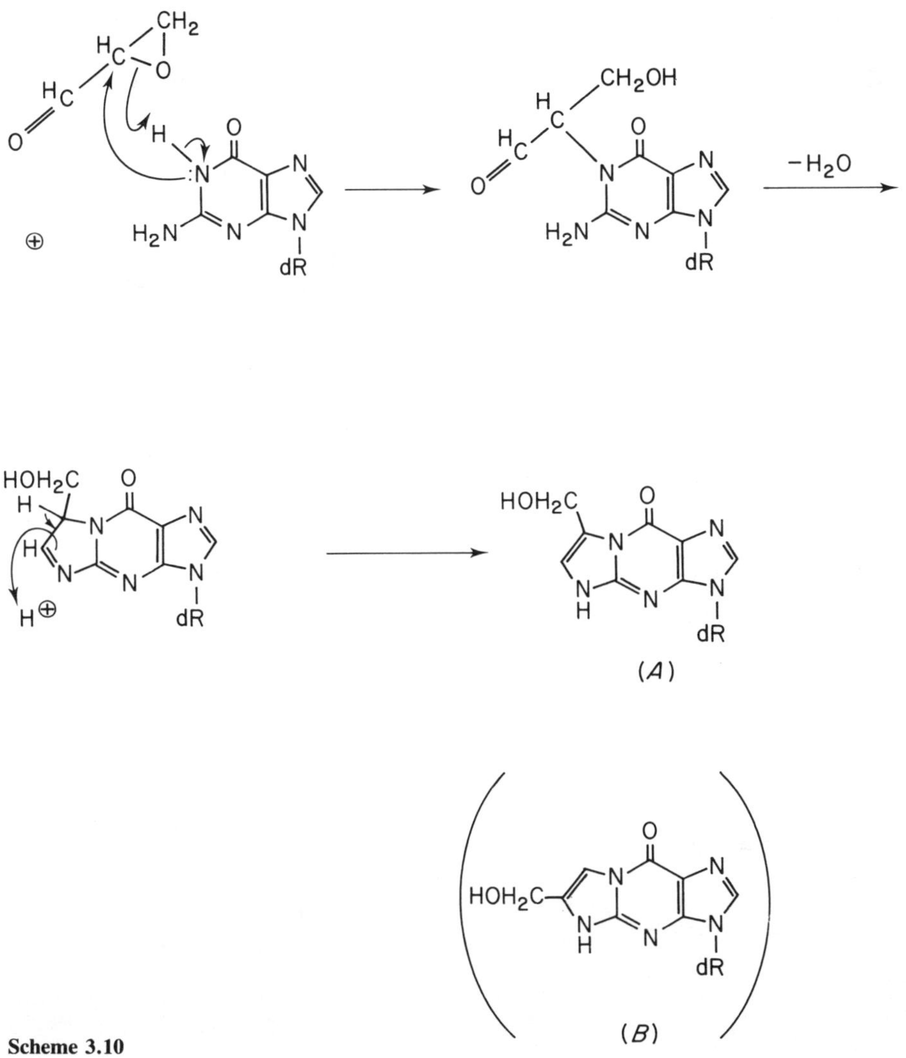

Scheme 3.10

alkylating function reacts with deoxyguanosine at weakly alkaline pH to bring about imidazo cyclization between the N-1 position and the C-2 amino group (Goldschmidt, Balzej and Van Duuren, 1968; Van Duuren, 1969). Whilst Van Duuren and his coworkers (Goldschmidt, Balzej and Van Duuren, 1968) did not identify their reaction product and proposed the alternative formulae (A) and (B) (*Scheme 3.10*), irrespective of the exact structure, bimolecular alkylation at the ring-nitrogen would appear to occur initially (*Scheme 3.10*). Imidazo cyclization would appear to account for glycidaldehyde mutagenicity (Corbett, Heidelberger and Dove, 1970; Izard, 1973; McCann *et al.*, 1975) and carcinogenicity in rodents (Van Duuren, Orris and Nelson, 1965; Van Duuren *et al.*, 1966, 1967a,b) as well as possibly for the carcinogenicity in rodents of glycidyl esters (Swern *et al.*, 1970).

Aflatoxins

An S_N2 mechanism would seem to apply also to reaction of aflatoxin B_1-2,3-epoxide (23) (*Scheme 3.11*) with DNA (and RNA). The structure of the DNA- and rRNA-bound adducts, obtained by Lin, Miller and Miller (1977) from the incubation of aflatoxin B_1 with, respectively, salmon-sperm DNA or rat-liver rRNA plus fortified hamster- or rat-liver microsomes, was deduced by hydrolysis, which gave 2,3-dihydro-2-(7-guanyl)-3-hydroxyaflatoxin B_1 (24) as the major product and 2,3-dihydro-2-[2,3,6-triamino-4-oxopyrimidin-N^5-yl)-*N*-formyl]-3-hydroxyaflatoxin B_1 (25) as a minor one. It was concluded that chemical reaction

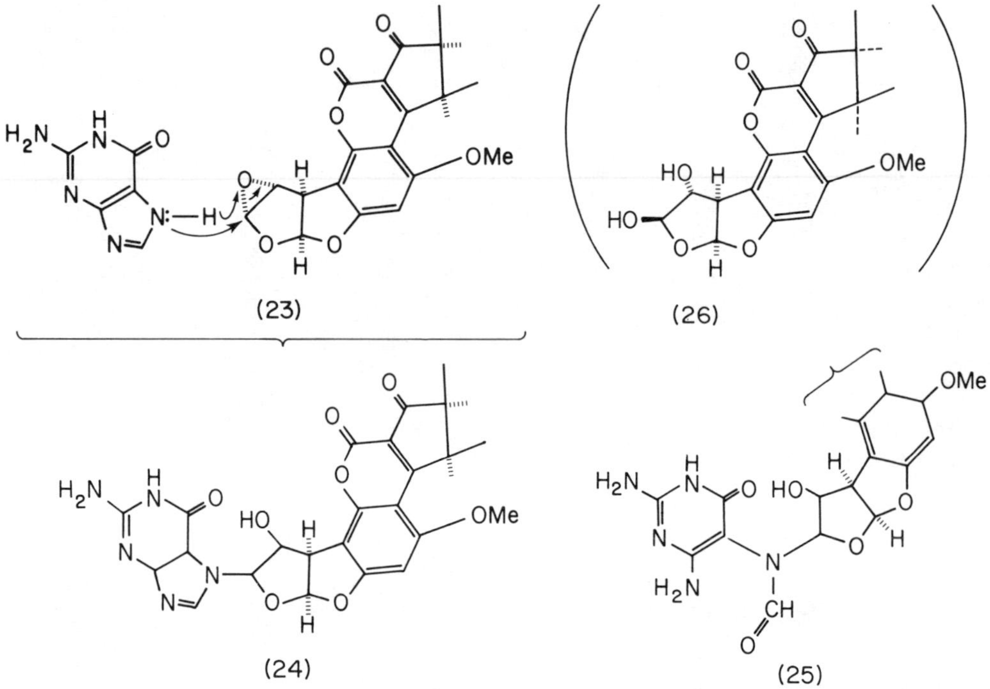

Scheme 3.11

had occurred therefore, both *in vitro* and *in vivo*, between the 2-position of aflatoxin B_1-2,3-epoxide (23) and N-7 of the DNA or RNA guanine residues. Biochemical investigation (Lin *et al.*, 1978) showed subsequently 2,3-dihydro-2,3-dihydroxyaflatoxin B_1 (26) to be a major aflatoxin B_1 metabolite in the presence of hamster- or rat-liver microsomes *in vitro*, but negligible amounts of (26) appeared to be formed in the presence of DNA. This result substantiated the biotransformation of aflatoxin B_1 in hamster and rat liver into aflatoxin B_1-2,3-epoxide, which would be expected to yield compound (26) on hydrolysis.

Garner *et al.* (1979) identified the major aflatoxin G_1–DNA adduct, which was formed both *in vitro* and *in vivo* and after peracid oxidation, and have shown it to be the *trans*-9,10-dihydro-9-(7-guanyl)-10-hydroxyaflatoxin G_1 (27). Thus, (27) is analogous to (24), which had been obtained in precisely the same way from aflatoxin B_1.

(27)

Polycyclic aromatic hydrocarbons

The interaction of the reactive metabolites of polycyclic aromatic hydrocarbons with nucleic acids has been the subject of a great deal of work (Phillips and Sims, 1979), much of which is exemplified by reference to that relating to benzo[a]pyrene.

In what appears to the present writer to have been key experiments, Meehan and Straub (1979) resolved (±)7β,8α-dihydroxy-9α,10α-epoxy-7,8,9,10-tetrahydrobenzo[a]pyrene, i.e. (±)*anti*-BP diol-epoxide, and reacted the optically pure (+) and (−)-enantiomers with native, calf-thymus DNA.

In *Scheme 3.12* are shown the deoxyguanosine residues in DNA which have reacted stereoselectively with *anti*-BP diol-epoxide racemate, so that the ratio of adduct obtained from the (+)-enantiomer to that from the (−)-enantiomer was 20:1, whereas the corresponding deoxyadenosine residues gave an almost identical distribution of deoxyadenosine diastereomeric products from the (+) and (−)-enantiomers. Meehan and Straub (1979) showed that the same ratio of diastereomers resulted through reaction of the separate enantiomers with native calf-thymus DNA. The exocyclic amino groups of the deoxyguanosine and deoxyadenosine residues were the sites of covalent binding concerned. This work demonstrated that the asymmetrical binding of the two enantiomeric *anti*-BP diol-epoxides to the exocyclic amino group of guanine in double-stranded DNA depends on the secondary structure of the polymer, as the two enantiomers reacted equally with the same position in single-stranded DNA, and there seems to have been (Weinstein *et al.*, 1976) greater heterogenicity of RNA adducts than of the DNA ones. One explanation for the capacity of DNA secondary structure to distinguish between two enantiomers derives from a stereoselective interaction, possibly an intercalation. This intercalation would occur readily with the (+)-enantiomer, but not with its mirror image. On the other hand, the lack of any stereoselectivity with regard to adenine covalent binding sites of double- and single-stranded DNA suggests that reaction with the diastereomers concerned does not implicate physical interaction.

As the difference in the level of covalent binding of (+) and (−)*anti*-BP diol-epoxides with the N^2-deoxyguanosine site in native DNA (Meehan and Straub, 1979) parallels the difference in mutagenic activity between (+) and (−)*anti*-BP diol-epoxides in a mammalian tissue-culture cell line (Wood *et al.*, 1977), and as (+)*anti*-BP diol-epoxide is the most carcinogenic of the four possible

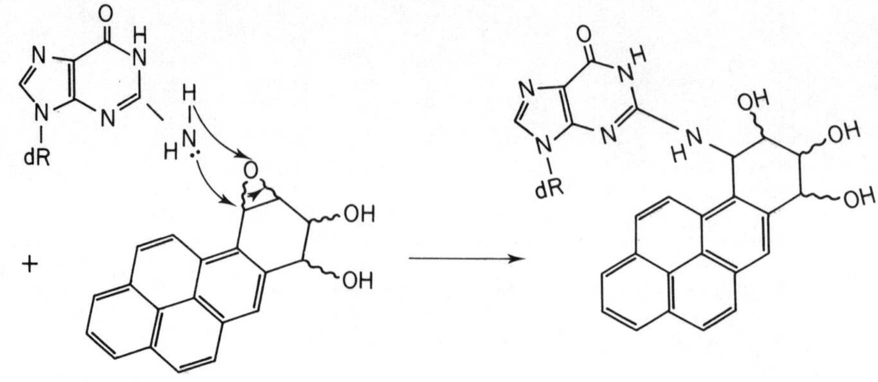

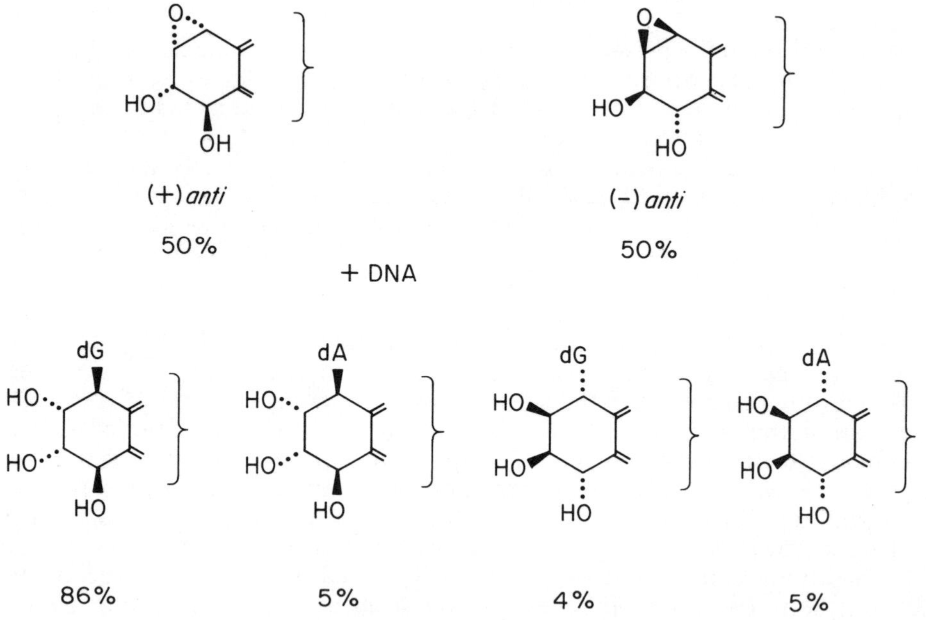

62 *Authenticated interactions with nucleic acid*

Scheme 3.12

(+) and (−)*anti*- and (+) and (−)*syn*-isomers in newborn mice (Buening *et al.*, 1978), the extent of this chemical (non-enzymic) reaction between (+)*anti*-BP diol-epoxide and double-stranded DNA correlates both with the mutagenic activity and with the tumorogenic potency. By corollary, Meehan and Straub's data (1979) seem to infer that any attempt to evaluate the carcinogenic potential of a polycyclic aromatic hydrocarbon ought to take account of the metabolic activation into putative carcinogenic intermediates and of their chemical and physical interactions

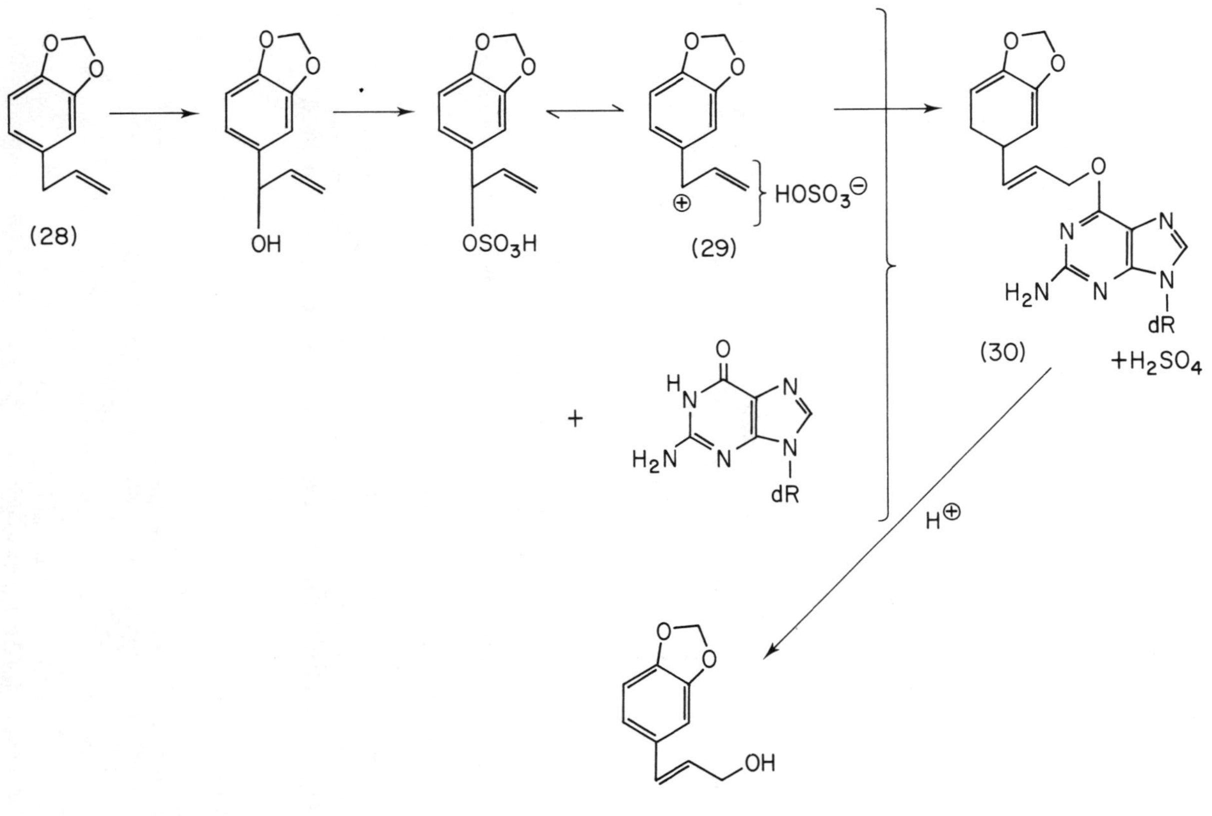

Scheme 3.13

with native DNA. High chemical reactivity of *anti-* and *syn-*BP diol-epoxide racemates probably accounts for a relative lack of carcinogenicity towards the skin of adult mice (Phillips and Sims, 1979).

Safrole

The reactive form of safrole (28) (*Scheme 3.13*), safrole-1'-sulphate (29), reacts both *in vitro* and *in vivo* with deoxyguanosine residues of hepatocyte DNA to yield O^6-(isosafrol-3'-yl)deoxyguanosine (30), which was characterized by n.m.r. spectroscopy (Borchert *et al.*, 1973) and mild acid degradation, which gave 3'-hydroxyisosafrole (31) (Wislocki *et al.*, 1976). The reaction between compound (29), which is a benzilic ester, and the deoxyguanosine residues is best described by the S_N1 mechanism (Hathway and Kolar, 1980) that is represented in *Scheme 3.13*.

Concluding remarks

This chapter stresses those interactions of reactive carcinogen metabolites with somatic DNA which would affect replication. There is a strong supposition that chemical reaction of small molecular alkylating agents, of epoxides, of hydroxylamines and their esters, or of benzilic esters with somatic DNA *in vivo* represents an initiating biochemical lesion (Peters, 1963), which belongs to the cancer causative mechanism. This proposition is examined at the beginning of the next chapter, which deals with the biological significance of these reactions in connection with DNA repair and miscoding during replication, and which pursues the predictability of mutation/carcinogenesis on this basis.

The role of secondary structure of the DNA helix in biological recognition processes has been mentioned briefly. It seems to be involved with the selection of (*a*) the enantiomers of *anti-*BP diol-epoxide racemate, and (*b*) reactive nucleophilic sites in DNA, the N-1 atom of adenine, for example, being greatly suppressed in fully H-bonded structures.

Finally, reference has been made to the role of polypeptides/proteins as ligands for the transport of reactive carcinogen electrophiles to the nuclei, and of cysteinyl peptides for detoxication of some reactive amino-azo dye metabolites.

Bibliography and references

BAKAY, B. and SOROF, S. (1964) *Cancer Res.*, **24**, 1814
BAKAY, B., SOROF, S. and SIEBERT, G. (1969) *Cancer Res.*, **29**, 23
BARBIN, A., BARTSCH, H., LECONTE, P. and RADMAN, M. (1981) *Nucleic Acid Res.*, **9**, 375
BARRIO, J.R., SECRIST, J.A. and LEONARD, N.J. (1972) *Biochem. Biophys. Res. Commun.*, **46**, 597
BARTSCH, H., MARGINSON, G.P., MALAVEILLE, C., CAMUS, A.M., BRUN, G., MARGINSON, J.M. *et al.* (1977) *Arch. Toxikol.*, **39**, 51
BECK, D.J. and BRUBAKER, R.R. (1975) *Mutat. Res.*, **27**, 181
BERWARD, Y. and SACHS, L. (1965) *J. Natl Cancer Inst.*, **35**, 641
BORCHERT, P., WISLOCKI, P.G., MILLER, J.A. and MILLER, E.C. (1973) *Cancer Res.*, **33**, 575
BUENING, M.K., WISLOCKI, P.G., LEVIN, W., YAGI, H., THAKKER, D.R., AKAGI, H. *et al.* (1978) *Proc. Natl Acad. Sci. USA*, **75**, 5358
CORBETT, T.H., HEIDELBERGER, C. and DOVE, W.F. (1970) *Mol. Pharmacol.*, **6**, 667
CRADDOCK, V.M. (1973) *Biochim. Biophys. Acta*, **312**, 202
DE BAUN, J.R., MILLER, E.C. and MILLER, J.A. (1970) *Cancer Res.*, **30**, 577

FREI, J.V. and LAWLEY, P.D. (1976) *Chem.-Biol. Interact.*, **13**, 215
GARNER, R.C., MARTIN, C.N., SMITH, J.R.L., COLES, B.F. and TOLSON, M.R. (1979) *Chem.-Biol. Interact.*, **26**, 57
GOLDSCHMIDT, B.M., BALZEJ, T.P. and VAN DUUREN, B.L. (1968) *Tetrahedron Lett.*, 1583
GOODGAME, D.M.L., JEEVES, I., PHILLIPS, F.L. and SKAPSKI, A.C. (1975) *Biochim. Biophys. Acta*, **378**, 153
GOTH, R. and RAJEWSKY, M.F. (1974a) *Proc. Natl Acad. Sci. USA*, **71**, 639
GOTH, R. and RAJEWSKY, M.F. (1974b) *Z. Krebsforschung*, **82**, 37
GREEN, T. and HATHWAY, D.E. (1978) *Chem.-Biol. Interact.*, **22**, 211
HALL, J.A., SAFFHILL, R., GREEN, T. and HATHWAY, D.E. (1981) *Carcinogenesis*, **2**, 141
HATHWAY, D.E. (1977) *Environ. Hlth Perspect.*, **21**, 55
HATHWAY, D.E. (1980) *Chem. Soc. Rev.*, **9**(1), 63
HATHWAY, D.E. and KOLAR, G.F. (1980) *Chem. Soc. Rev.*, **9**(2), 241
INTERNATIONAL AGENCY FOR RESEARCH ON CANCER (1979) *Monographs on the Evaluation of the Carcinogenic Risk to Humans: Some Monomers, Plastics and Synthetic Elastomers and Acrolein.* Vol. 19, pp. 377–438. Lyon, France: IARC
IZARD, M.C. (1973) *C.R. Hebd. Séances Acad. Sci., Paris*, **276**, 3037
KADLUBAR, F.F., MILLER, J.A. and MILLER, E.C. (1978) *Cancer Res.*, **38**, 3628
KETTERER, B., KADLUBAR, F.F., FLAMMANG, T., CARNE, T. and ENDERBY, G. (1979) *Chem.-Biol. Interact.*, **25**, 7
KETTERER, B., TIPPING, E., BEALE, D., MEUWISSEN, J. and KAY, C.M. (1975) In *Chemical and Viral Oncogenesis. Proceedings of the Xth International Cancer Congress.* Eds P. Bucalossi, U. Veronesi and N. Cascinelli. Vol. 2, pp. 25–29. New York: American Elsevier Publ. Co.
KLEIHUES, P., KOLAR, G.F. and MARGINSON, G.P. (1976) *Cancer Res.*, **36**, 2189
KOPELOVICH, L., CONLON, S. and POLLACK, R. (1977) *Proc. Natl Acad. Sci. USA*, **74**, 3019
KRIEK, E. (1972) *Cancer Res.*, **32**, 2042
KRIEK, E. (1974) *Biochim. Biophys. Acta*, **355**, 177
KRIEK, E. and HENGEVELD, G.M. (1978) *Chem.-Biol. Interact.*, **21**, 179
KRIEK, E., MILLER, J.A., JUHL, U. and MILLER, E.C. (1967) *Biochemistry*, **6**, 177
LAIB, R.J. and BOLT, H.M. (1977) *Toxicology*, **8**, 185
LAIB, R.J. and BOLT, H.M. (1978) *Arch. Toxicol.*, **39**, 235
LAWLEY, P.D. (1974) *Mutat. Res.*, **23**, 283
LAWLEY, P.D. (1976) In *Screening Tests in Chemical Carcinogenesis.* Eds R. Montesano, H. Bartsch and L. Tomatis. International Agency for Research on Cancer Scientific Publications no. 12, pp. 181–208. Lyon, France: IARC
LECOINTE, P., MACQUET, J.-P., BUTOUR, J.-L. and PAOLETTI, C. (1977) *Mutat. Res.*, **48**, 139
LIN, J.-K., JENNAN, K.A., MILLER, E.C. and MILLER, J.A. (1978) *Cancer Res.*, **38**, 2424
LIN, J.-K., MILLER, J.A. and MILLER, E.C. (1977) *Cancer Res.*, **37**, 4430
LITWACK, G., KETTERER, B. and ARIAS, I.M. (1971) *Nature*, **234**, 466
McCANN, J., CHOI, E., YAMASAKI, E. and AMES, B.N. (1975) *Proc. Natl Acad. Sci. USA*, **72**, 5135
MAINIGI, K.D. and SOROF, S. (1977) *Proc. Natl Acad. Sci. USA*, **74**, 2293
MANSY, S., CHU, G.Y.H., DUNCAN, R.E. and TOBIAS, R.S. (1978) *J. Am. Chem. Soc.*, **100**, 607
MARGINSON, G.P., LIKHACHEV, A.J. and KOLAR, G.F. (1979) *Chem.-Biol. Interact.*, **25**, 345
MEEHAN, T. and STRAUB, K. (1979) *Nature*, **277**, 410
MILLER, J.A. and MILLER, E.C. (1947) *Cancer Res.*, **7**, 468
MILLER, J.A. and MILLER, E.C. (1969) *Prog. Exp. Tumor Res.*, **11**, 273
MILLER, J.A. and MILLER, E.C. (1971) *J. Natl Cancer Inst.*, **47**, v
MILLER, R.W. and TODARO, G.J. (1969) *Lancet*, **i**, 81
MONTI-BRAGADINI, C., TANARO, M. and BANFI, E. (1975) *Chem.-Biol. Interact.*, **11**, 469
NICOLL, J.M., SWANN, P.F. and PEGG, A.E. (1977) *Chem.-Biol. Interact.*, **16**, 301
O'CONNOR, P.J., CAPPS, M.J. and CRAIG, A.W. (1973) *Br. J. Cancer*, **27**, 153
OESCH, F. and DOERJER, G. (1982) *Carcinogenesis*, **3**, 663
PEGG, A.E. (1977) *Adv. Cancer Res.*, **25**, 195
PETERS, SIR RUDOLPH (1963) *Biochemical Lesions and Lethal Synthesis.* Oxford: Pergamon Press
PHILLIPS, D.H. and SIMS, P. (1979) In *Chemical Carcinogens and DNA.* Ed. P.L. Grover. Vol. 2, pp. 29–58. Boca Raton, Florida: CRC Press
ROBERTS, J.J. and THOMSON, A.J. (1979) *Prog. Nucleic Acid Res. Mol. Biol.*, **22**, 71
ROBINS, A.B. (1973) *Chem.-Biol. Interact.*, **6**, 35
SANI, B.P., MOTT, D.M., SZAJMAN, S.M. and SOROF, S. (1972) *Biochem. Biophys. Res. Commun.*, **49**, 1598
SATTSANGI, P.D., LEONARD, N.J. and FRIHART, C.R. (1977) *J. Org. Chem.*, **42**, 3296
SCRIBNER, J.D. and NAIMY, N.K. (1973) *Cancer Res.*, **33**, 1159
SCRIBNER, J.D. and NAIMY, N.K. (1975) *Cancer Res.*, **35**, 1416

SCRIBNER, N.K. and SCRIBNER, J.D. (1979) *Chem.-Biol. Interact.*, **26**, 47
SCRIBNER, N.K., SCRIBNER, J.D., SMITH, D.L., SCHRAM, K.H. and McCLOSKEY, J.A. (1979) *Chem.-Biol. Interact.*, **26**, 27
SINGER, B. (1975) *Prog. Nucleic Acid Res. Mol. Biol.*, **15**, 219
SOROF, S. and YOUNG, E.M. (1973) *Cancer Res.*, **33**, 2010
SOROF, S., YOUNG, E.M., McBRIDE, R.A. and COFFEY, C.B. (1970) *Cancer Res.*, **30**, 2029
SOROF, S., YOUNG, E.M., McCUE, M.M. and FETTERMAN, P.L. (1963) *Cancer Res.*, **23**, 864
SPENGLER, S. and SINGER, B. (1981) *Nucleic Acid Res.*, **9**, 365
SUN, L. and SINGER, B. (1975) *Biochemistry*, **14**, 1795
SWENSON, D.H., FARMER, P.D. and LAWLEY, P.D. (1976) *Chem.-Biol. Interact.*, **15**, 91
SWERN, D., WIEDER, R., McDONOGH, M., MERANZE, D.R. and SHIMKIN, M.B. (1970) *Cancer Res.*, **30**, 1037
TOPAL, M.D. and FRESCO, J.R. (1976) *Nature*, **263**, 285
VAN DUUREN, B.L. (1969) *Ann. N.Y. Acad. Sci.*, **163**, 133
VAN DUUREN, B.L., LANGSETH, L., GOLDSCHMIDT, B.M. and ORRIS, L. (1967a) *J. Natl Cancer Inst.*, **39**, 1217
VAN DUUREN, B.L., LANGSETH, L., ORRIS, L., BADEN, M. and KUSCHNER, M. (1967b) *J. Natl Cancer Inst.*, **39**, 1213
VAN DUUREN, B.L., LANGSETH, L., ORRIS, L., TEEBOR, G., NELSON, N. and KUSCHNER, M. (1966) *J. Natl Cancer Inst.*, **37**, 825
VAN DUUREN, B.L., ORRIS, L. and NELSON, N. (1965) *J. Natl Cancer Inst.*, **35**, 707
WANG, A.H.J., BARRIO, J.R. and PAUL, I.C. (1976) *J. Am. Chem. Soc.*, **98**, 7401
WANG, A.H.J., DAMMAN, L.G., BARRIO, J.R. and PAUL, I.C. (1974) *J. Am. Chem. Soc.*, **96**, 1205
WEINSTEIN, I.B., JEFFREY, A.M., JENETTE, K.W., BLOBSTEIN, S.H., HARVEY, R.G., HARRIS, C. et al. (1976) *Science*, **193**, 592
WESTRA, J.G., KRIEK, E. and HITTENHAUSEN, H. (1976) *Chem.-Biol. Interact.*, **15**, 149
WISLOCKI, P.G., BORCHERT, P., MILLER, J.A. and MILLER, E.C. (1976) *Cancer Res.*, **36**, 1686
WOOD, A.W., CHANG, R.L., LEVIN, W., YAGI, H., THAKKER, D.R., JERINA, D.M. et al. (1977) *Biochem. Biophys. Res. Commun.*, **77**, 1389

Chapter 4

Mechanisms in perspective: biological significance of modified deoxyribonucleoside residues in DNA

At this stage in the narrative, the proposition that 'highly active chemical carcinogen intermediates react with target-organ DNA in such a way that effects somatic mutation' appears to be consistent with the fact that:

(a) Chemical carcinogens promote the induction of tumours in experimental mammals (Chapter 2).
(b) A relationship involving dose and time applies to carcinogenic potency (Druckrey and Küpfmüller, 1948; Jones and Grendon, 1975).
(c) Chemical carcinogens *per se* undergo metabolic activation in the mammal (Chapter 2).
(d) In turn, highly reactive, carcinogen-derived electrophiles react specifically with somatic DNA (Chapter 3).
(e) Chemical carcinogens in the presence of a metabolically activating system, and reactive carcinogen intermediates directly, behave as mutagens (Chapter 2).
(f) Chemical carcinogens transform normal cells into tumour cells (Chapter 3).
(g) Specific chemicals inhibit or prevent the induction of tumours by chemical carcinogens (Chapter 5).
(h) Other substances, known as promoters, increase the potency of weak carcinogens (Chapter 6).

The foregoing statements were obtained by experiment and inductive reasoning, and 'they may be considered to be true or very nearly true until (a) they are corrected and made more accurate by further observations (or experimentation), or (b) they are shown to have exceptions' (Newton's fourth rule of reasoning in philosophy).

An additional contribution to the basic problem is made in Chapters 4–6 of this book, essentially by following Newton's method (q.v.).

The present chapter has to do with the biological significance of specific interactions by carcinogen-related intermediates with deoxyribonucleoside residues of DNA. Relevant researches explore the persistence of these biochemical lesions vis-à-vis DNA repair, the miscoding induced during DNA-directed DNA biosynthesis, and the effects on the biosynthesis of DNA and other macromolecules.

Repair of biochemical lesions in DNA

It ought to be clearly stated at the outset of this discussion that precise mechanisms have yet to be established for DNA repair processes. In reality, only the persistence in DNA of modified DNA components, themselves isotopically labelled from work with labelled carcinogens, has been monitored, and the evidence at first sight is often difficult to understand. Interpretation of the persistence of labelled DNA components, and conversely of its elimination in terms of an excision mechanism, derives from an assimilation of all of the relevant data and from supporting enzymic studies.

In the section of Chapter 3 that is concerned with N-nitrosamines and 3-alkyl-1-phenyltriazenes, it became evident that, out of all the possible alkylations of the deoxyribonucleoside residues of DNA, the degree of O^6-alkylation of the deoxyguanosine residues correlates best with the overall carcinogenic potency of these chemical carcinogens (Loveless, 1969), and this modification of DNA emerges as the most probable miscoding biochemical lesion in these cases. The fact that the highest degree of O^6-alkylation matched the tissue specificities of the MNU (Kleihues and Magee, 1973; Goth and Rajewsky, 1974a) and MPT (Bartsch et al., 1977) carcinogens seems to mirror the very simple cases of Me-N_2^+ generation involved (q.v.) and, in general, additional factors may have to be taken into account. Different biological situations are presented where stable intermediates function as transport forms (Druckrey et al., 1967). Particular importance attaches to the operation of DNA-repair processes, as (a) work with rats, exposed to DMN, showed a rapid loss of O^6-methylguanine from the liver DNA (O'Connor, Capps and Craig, 1973), (b) in general, the highest concentration of O^6-alkylguanine in DNA in vivo does not necessarily parallel the tissue specificities of the alkylating carcinogens in question, and (c) intact Escherichia coli DNA after treatment with MNNG also showed a rapid loss of O^6-methylguanine in vivo (Lawley and Orr, 1970).

In fact, the tissue with the greatest susceptibility towards the induction of tumours by a specific alkylating carcinogen is one in which the repair process for the corresponding O^6-alkylation of the deoxyguanosine residues in the DNA is least efficient (see also Chapter 2). Low turnover of these promutagenic lesions in DNA would at any rate contribute to the probability of the occurrence of miscoding events during DNA biosynthesis and, thus, would predispose the tissue in question to malignancy. A great deal of work on the persistence of modified DNA components in tissue DNA in vivo, and by corollary on the excision mechanism, has been made with the alkylations by N-nitroso compounds (see also Pegg, 1977b; Margison and O'Connor, 1979; O'Connor, Saffhill and Margison, 1979). The progress made adumbrates that with other chemical carcinogens, and this is reflected in the present narrative.

In agreement with the foregoing argument, it was found that, after administration of such a (single) dose of ENU to newborn rats as was known to produce a high incidence of c.n.s. tumours, the extent of O^6-ethylation of the deoxyguanosine residues in the DNA of all of the tissues that were investigated was essentially similar, but that loss of O^6-ethylation of the brain DNA was much slower than from non-target organ DNA (Goth and Rajewsky, 1974b). Again, a spate of work in different sensitive species of animal (Kleihues and Margison, 1974; Nicoll, Swann and Pegg, 1975; Lawley, 1976; Margison, Margison and Montesano, 1976; Cox and Irving, 1977; Kleihues and Bücheler, 1977; Likhachev, Margison and Montesano, 1977; Frei et al., 1978; Margison, Likhachev and Kolar, 1979; Swenberg et al., 1979) also showed that O^6-alkylguanine persisted for a far longer period of time in the DNA of tissues susceptible to tumour induction than in that of non-target tissues, but complicating factors operated in some other cases. Thus, in two strains of mouse with different susceptibilities to the induction of DMN liver tumours, the liver DNA was methylated to a similar extent (Den Engelse, 1974), but the proliferative response, measured in terms of DNA synthesis, was much more extensive in the susceptible than in the resistant-strain hepatocytes (De Munter, Den Engelse and Emmelot, 1979). Again, the dosing of rats on a repetitive schedule respectively with DMPT (Cooper et al., 1978) and DMN (Nicoll, Swann and Pegg, 1977) produced the highest level of O^6-methylguanine in the brain DNA in the case of DMPT and in kidney DNA in that of DMN: the target organs for the two alkylating carcinogens. On the other hand, the chronic treatment of rats by repeated small doses of DMN, which is specific for the induction of hepatomas, led to the retention of O^6-methylguanine in the kidney and lung DNA and to its loss from liver DNA (Margison, Margison and Montesano, 1977), because this hepatocarcinogenic regimen accelerated the already considerable rate of elimination of O^6-methylguanine from hepatic DNA (Kleihues and Margison, 1976; Margison, Margison and Montesano, 1977; Nicoll, Swann and Pegg, 1977). Thus, the elimination of this purine analogue, viz. O^6-methylguanine, from liver DNA is strongly (DMN) dose dependent (Kleihues and Margison, 1976; Pegg, 1977a).

The following empirical observations support the foregoing proposition. For example, the elimination of O^6-methylguanine from DNA is accelerated by chronic treatment with various chemical compounds (Pegg, 1977a,b; Cooper et al., 1978), but the loss of O^6-methylguanine from DNA, caused by low doses of DMN or MNU, is inhibited by prior treatment with relatively higher doses of the same agent (Kleihues and Margison, 1976; Pegg, 1977a; Pegg and Hui, 1978a) or with other substances which react with DNA (Kleihues and Margison, 1976; Pegg, 1978a). A single large dose of DMN was found (Pegg and Hui, 1978b) to inhibit temporarily the DNA repair of the O^6-methyldeoxyguanosine lesions that were formed by the same treatment.

Pegg (1977b) argued the physiological consequences of the underlying proposition (see above). Thus, if small amounts of O^6-methylguanine, produced in DNA by exposure to very low levels of DMN, may be repaired efficiently, then this DNA-repair mechanism might protect against (DMN) carcinogenesis. The foregoing argument would be consistent with the presence in the working environment of a chemical plant for the responsible manufacture of an industrial chemical which is a frank carcinogen, of only very low concentrations, and with the fact that the operatives do not contract cancer from this source. It follows that a threshold dose of DMN may be defined as that dose at which the rate of DNA methylation is very similar to that of DNA repair. Doses below this threshold level would not be expected to cause a significant increase in the induction of liver tumours. The following experimental facts are relevant. Whilst exposure to 20 ppm of DMN in the diet without limit caused liver cancer in 66% of the rats, exposure to 5 ppm of DMN in the diet produced only an 8% incidence of cancer (Terracini, Magee and Barnes, 1967). Since these dietary levels of DMN correspond to the dose level at which elimination of O^6-methylguanine from DNA was more efficient after lower doses, the levels of this purine analogue in liver DNA appear to be therefore disproportionately greater than after the higher dose. Even exposure to

2 ppm of DMN in the diet caused one tumour in one out of 37 animals, and the threshold dose must be below this level of intake but, on the other hand, no hepatomas have ever been produced by a single dose of DMN or MNU in normal adult rats (Terracini, Magee and Barnes, 1967).

The induction and inhibition of the DNA-repair process for the O^6-methyldeoxyguanosine lesion (*see above*) suggests that the process which operates for repair of O^6-methylguanine may extend also to:

(a) The repair of higher O^6-alkylguanine lesions (Craddock, 1975a,b; Kleihues and Margison, 1976; Pegg, 1977a, 1978a).
(b) Other types of DNA modification (Kleihues and Margison, 1976).

With regard to mechanisms, *E. coli* endonuclease II excises O^6-methylguanine (as well as 3-methyladenine, N^2-substituted adenines and N^2-substituted guanines) from modified DNA *in vitro* (Kirtikar and Goldthwait, 1974; Kirtikar, Dipple and Goldthwait, 1975), and leaves apurinic sites. In such a system, there is no possibility of the occurrence of O-demethylation without any excision. The feasible operation of this mechanism in mammals, followed by limited further digestion of the 'nicked' DNA strand and subsequent DNA repair synthesis and ligase action, would correspond to the 'short repair' system observed in mammals after the action of ionizing radiation and certain alkylating agents (Regan and Setlow, 1974; Cleaver, 1975). When the cytosol from various rat tissues was incubated with DNA that had undergone a low degree of MNU methylation, however, no O^6-methylguanine was liberated (Pegg, 1978b). This suggests the unlikelihood of the adoption of the endonuclease II depurination by mammalian cells *in vivo*, and the liberation of methanol implicates O-demethylation (Pegg, 1978b). Two systems may operate in the removal of O^6-methylguanine from DNA in rats, as more of that formed in liver DNA by low doses of DMN was removed than of that formed by higher doses; this suggests that one system may be saturated by small amounts of this purine analogue, whereas a less efficient system may possess much greater capacity for effecting its removal (Pegg, 1977a; Pegg and Hui, 1978b). Amongst the previously mentioned experiments in sensitive species of animal concerning the operation of DNA repair, there were those made in Syrian golden hamsters (Margison, Margison and Montesano, 1976). Their relevance in the present connotation relates to the fact that the rate of elimination of O^6-methylguanine from hepatic DNA after higher dose levels of DMN is much slower in Syrian golden hamsters than in rats (Margison, Margison and Montesano, 1976; Stumpf *et al.*, 1979), although it is rapidly eliminated after low doses in both species. The marked species difference was held (Margison, Margison and Montesano, 1976; Stumpf *et al.*, 1979) to be consistent with the species specificity that is shown to the induction of DMN tumours, i.e. to the greater sensitivity of the hamster liver.

Other work deals with the elimination from DNA of other alkylation products, formed by *N*-nitroso compounds in mammalian cells and bacteria. This seems to be less relevant to tumour induction by alkylating agents, however, than that relating to DNA repair after O^6-alkylation of the deoxyguanosine residues for, unlike the corresponding O^6-alkylguanosine analogues, other alkylated purine (and pyrimidine) analogues are less likely to be involved with miscoding events (*see above*). Nevertheless, brief reference ought to be made to this work as (a) the very nature of some of the results *per se* strongly supports the arguments with regard to a DNA-repair process for O^6-alkylguanine, and (b) some of them may be germane to the specific interactions that have been found between reactive metabolites of the more structurally complex carcinogens and DNA (Chapter 3).

In general, alkylation by N-nitroso compounds affords preponderating 7-alkylation of deoxyguanosine residues of DNA besides the corresponding O^6-alkylations (Chapter 3), which have been the subject of this discussion hitherto. Elimination of the former seems to occur at essentially similar rates in all of the organs of the rat, provided the appropriate allowance be made for loss due to cell death at higher doses of carcinogen, and for the ionic strength and pH of the nuclear environment (Margison et al., 1973; Goth and Rajewsky, 1974a; Pegg and Nicoll, 1976). At any rate in rat liver, the rates of elimination of 7-methylguanine from DNA in vitro and in vivo are strictly similar (Craddock, 1969). Accordingly, these findings mitigate against an active excision mechanism for the elimination of 7-alkylguanine. Additional evidence against active excision arises from the absence of effect of the stage in the cell cycle on the rate of elimination of 7-alkylguanine from DNA. Thus, no increase in rate of elimination was caused through the hyperplasia stimulated by partial hepatectomy (Capps, O'Connor and Craig, 1973), compared with the steady state in resting liver (Margison et al., 1973). It might be said that the degree of 7-alkylation of the deoxyguanosine residues of DNA is independent of the chemical properties, tumorigenic potency and tissue specificities of the alkylating agent (Schoental, 1967; Swann and Magee, 1968, 1971; Goth and Rajewsky, 1972; Kleihues and Magee, 1973). In the absence of an excision mechanism for 7-alkylguanines, the possibility of modifying such activity by high doses of carcinogen or its chronic administration does not arise. Other work (Frei and Lawley, 1975; Margison, Margison and Montesano, 1976) has shown that the rates of elimination of 7-alkyladenines from mammalian DNA in vitro and in vivo were strictly similar, and indicated the absence of an excision mechanism for the 7-adenine analogues. Finally, as 7-alkylpurines are not miscoding bases in DNA, a defence mechanism for their active elimination may be unnecessary in respect of exposed mammals.

The rate of elimination of 3-alkyladenines from the DNA of mammalian cells compared with that of spontaneous depurination (Margison and O'Connor, 1973; Goth and Rajewsky, 1974a,b; Kleihues and Margison, 1974; Craddock, 1975b; Frei and Lawley, 1975; Margison, Margison and Montesano, 1976) provided good evidence for the occurrence of an enzymic mechanism of excision for these adenine analogues. E. coli endonuclease II (see above) reacted more rapidly with 3-methyladenine in DNA than with the O^6-methylguanine (Kirtikar and Goldthwait, 1974) and the rate of elimination of the adenine analogue was faster in vivo than in vitro. In mammals, however, as the rate of elimination of 3-alkyladenines from cerebral DNA is very much faster than that of O^6-alkylguanines (Goth and Rajewsky, 1974a; Kleihues and Margison, 1974), these activities must be separate, at any rate in brain cells. Again, unlike the excision of O^6-methylguanine from DNA, 3-methyladenine excision cannot be induced or inhibited either by high doses or by chronic administration of carcinogens, and the enzymic activity of the excision mechanism shows little variability between the tissues (Pegg and Hui, 1978a).

In rats treated chronically with MNU, 3-methylguanine was found in cerebral DNA, but not in non-target organ DNA, and this observation was attributed to a deficiency in the excision mechanism for this guanine analogue, which permitted its accumulation in the brain (Margison and Kleihues, 1975). 3-Methylguanine was excised also from the liver DNA of Syrian golden hamsters administered DMN (Margison, Margison and Montesano, 1976).

Hence, much of the present evidence is indicative of an enzymic mechanism for the elimination from DNA of 3-alkylpurines.

In comparison with the work on the repair of alkylated lesions in DNA, which has been the subject of this section hitherto, scant attention has been paid (McElhone, O'Connor and Craig, 1971; Margison, Margison and Montesano, 1979) to the feasible repair of alkylated lesions in RNA.

Straightforward evidence revealed that DNA is the principal target site for neutral platinum complexes in mammals (Chapter 3) and that the interactions with DNA impair its function as template for DNA replication (Roberts and Thomson, 1979) (*see below*). The biochemical lesions in question are recognized by an excision–repair process and removed (Van den Berg and Roberts, 1975a,b), and furthermore both they and the excision–repair machinery are recognized in turn by a caffeine-sensitive process (Roberts and Ward, 1973), which appears to facilitate the capacity of the replicating process to synthesize (DNA) past them (Van den Berg and Roberts, 1975a; Fravall and Roberts, 1978).

Persistence studies as such have not been made in the case of vinyl chloride-induced angiosarcoma of the liver. In a 2-year experiment, however, in which rats had been exposed to unlabelled vinyl chloride in their drinking water (250 ppm), the presence of imidazo-cyclization products of the deoxycytidine and deoxyadenosine residues of target-organ DNA was detected in surviving animals up to and beyond the time of tumour induction (Green and Hathway, 1978). This evidence would appear to be consistent with the persistence of these modified deoxyribonucleoside residues in hepatic fibroblastic DNA and with the absence of an excision mechanism from the DNA of hepatic fibroblastic elements, and entirely irrespective of any hepatocyte excision mechanism.

Brookes and Lawley (1964) demonstrated the covalent binding of polycyclic aromatic hydrocarbons to DNA, RNA and proteins in mouse skin, and showed that the extent of the binding to mouse-skin DNA correlated strongly with the potency of these substances to induce skin tumours. Other workers (Lawley, 1966; Lieberman and Dipple, 1972; Rayman and Dipple, 1973) using model 7-bromomethylbenz[a]anthracenes showed this sort of persistence and correlation. Such evidence stresses the importance of that target-organ DNA to tumour induction. More recently, however, Phillips, Grover and Sims (1978) did not find any ready correlation between the carcinogenic effects of three polycyclic aromatic hydrocarbons in three strains of mouse which showed a marked strain specificity in their carcinogenic response, either with the extent of the reaction with DNA, or with the persistence of covalent binding with the deoxyribonucleoside residues of DNA.

It would appear that in these circumstances (Phillips, Grover and Sims, 1978), as was argued in the case of the simple alkylating agents, complicating factors interfere with the amount of bound nucleoside analogues in the tissue DNA and/or with the excision mechanism. These effects would be impossible to analyse, because of the unavailability of a corresponding background of inter-related information to that available for the interpretation of those phenomena in respect of an excision mechanism for alkylations by *N*-nitroso compounds. But, other factors may have been involved such as, for example, the physiological state of the tissue concerned, and reference might be made to *N*-nitrosamine alkylation (Margison, Margison and Montesano, 1977), which controls the degree of cell proliferation, and which may also determine the incidence of base-mispairing (mutagenic) events that occur in replicating DNA, and may even limit DNA replication.

Miscoding induced by carcinogens during directed nucleic acid biosynthesis

The evidence obtained by this method complements and confirms that resulting from investigation of DNA repair (*see above*). As it would be impossible to study the feasible misincorporations into DNA and RNA resulting from chemical carcinogens during replication *in vivo*, recourse has had to be made, for such experiments, to DNA and RNA-synthesizing systems *in vitro*, which utilize bacterial DNA and RNA polymerases acting on DNA-like or RNA-like templates that contain various proportions of the new analogues of the constituent (purine and pyrimidine) bases, which were formed through interaction with reactive carcinogen metabolite(s). This (molecular biological) method aims to explain the mutagenicity of such chemical carcinogens as have been tested in this way, on the assumption that specifically modified bases, like O^6-alkylguanine in the case of the *N*-nitroso compounds (Loveless, 1969), would interfere with the H-bonding of the (dA–dT) and (dC–dG) base-pairs in the Watson–Crick double helix for DNA (Lawley and Brookes, 1961; Kreig, 1963; Ludlum and Wilhelm, 1968; Singer and Fraenkel-Conrat, 1970; Lawley, Orr and Shah, 1971/1972; Lawley *et al.*, 1973; Singer, 1976). Templates, synthesized by polynucleotide phosphorylase from a relevant mixture of ribonucleoside diphosphates, contain one modified base. They are employed with RNA polymerase, and have been in use for a considerable period of time. On the other hand, the templates, prepared through the interaction of reactive carcinogen metabolites, clearly contain more than one modified base. These templates are used with DNA polymerase, and they have been in use only recently (Abbott and Saffhill, 1977a,b). The utilization of DNA polymerase is advantageous, as this enzyme system is associated with a very low natural error frequency (Loeb *et al.*, 1980), viz. about one error in 10^5, compared with RNA polymerase, Such an accuracy for the DNA polymerase system, taken in conjunction with the use of a double-stranded template, permits the detection of very low levels indeed of misincorporation arising from the presence of small amounts of miscoding base.

Both DNA-polymerase and RNA-polymerase systems have been used to detect miscodings induced by *N*-nitroso compounds in DNA and RNA biosynthesis *in vitro*. An early paper (Ludlum, 1970a) using RNA-directed RNA polymerase showed that 7-methylguanine pairs normally (like guanine) with cytosine, and that no mispairing with thymine occurred. This result was confirmed with DNA-directed DNA polymerase (Abbott and Saffhill, 1977b). Similarly, the methylated analogues, 7-methyladenine, 3-methyladenine and 3-methylguanine, 1-methyladenine and 3-methylthymine do not invoke miscoding in biosynthesis involving the DNA-directed DNA polymerase (Abbott and Saffhill, 1977a,b). (Cross-reference might be made here to the corresponding work on DNA-repair.) On the other hand, O^6-ethylguanine and O^6-methylguanine cause misincorporations in the two systems (Gerchman and Ludlum, 1973; Abbott and Saffhill, 1977b); cytosine does not pair with O^6-alkylguanine in the RNA-directed RNA-polymerase system. O^4-Methylthymine caused errors in the DNA-polymerase system, where miscoding was uncompetitive (Abbott and Saffhill, 1977a), and O^4-methyluracil caused errors in the RNA-polymerase system (Singer, Fraenkel-Conrat and Kúsmierck, 1978). Thus, O^4-alkylation of thymine and uracil are as important promutagenic lesions as O^6-alkylguanine is. An interesting

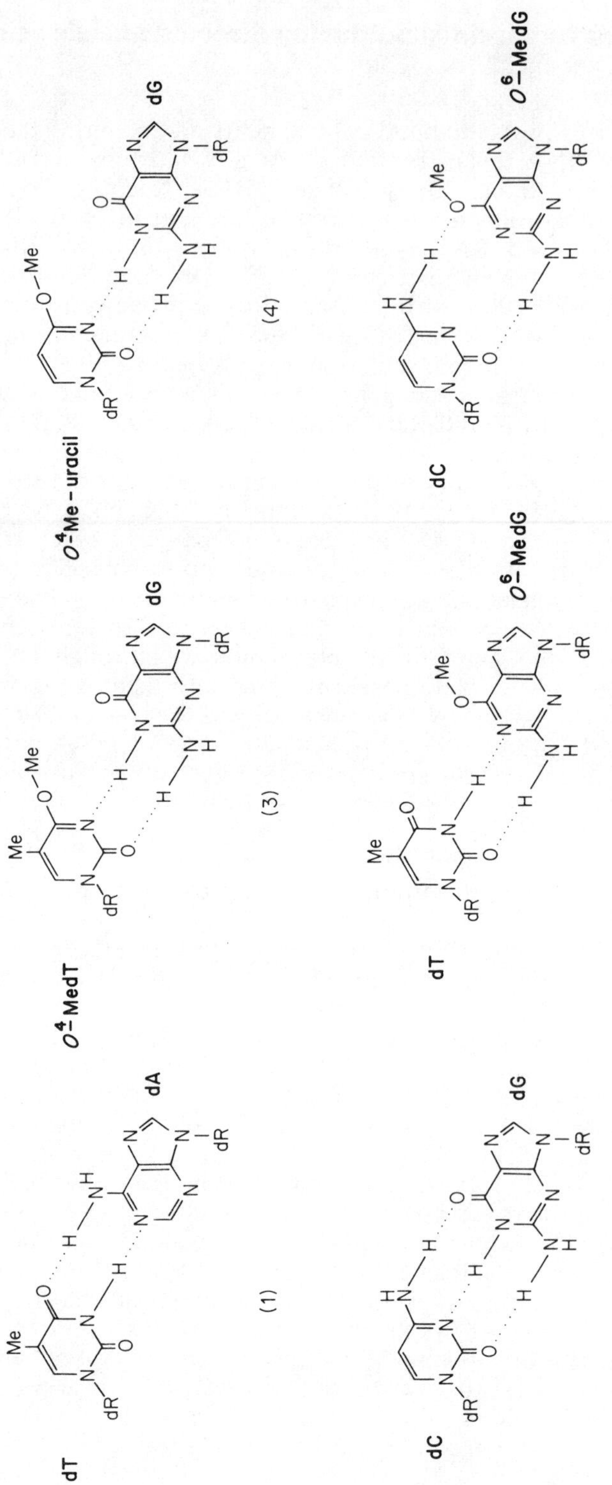
dT
dA
(1)
dC
dG
(2)
O⁴-MedT
dG
(3)
dT
O⁶-MedG
(5)
O⁴-Me-uracil
dG
(4)
dC
O⁶-MedG
(6)

Scheme 4.1

difference in behaviour of O^2-methylthymine, which pairs 'normally' with adenine in the case of DNA polymerase (Saffhill and Abbott, 1978), and which miscodes with guanine in the RNA-polymerase system (Singer, Fraenkel-Conrat and Kúsmierck, 1978), must be attributed to the enzyme specificities. The presence of phosphotriesters in DNA templates did not cause errors in DNA biosynthesis (Abbott and Saffhill, 1977a,b).

Thus, miscoding occurs only where it is possible to construct a stable, coplanar H-bonded base-pair (*Scheme 4.1*) (O'Connor, Saffhill and Margison, 1979). [In *Scheme 4.1*, the normal Watson–Crick dA–dT (1) and dC–dG (2) base-pairs have been included for reference.] Miscoding by O^4-methylthymine (3) and O^4-methyluracil (4) are readily understandable in terms of the H-bonded pairing with other bases. Similarly, the competitive nature of the miscoding of O^6-methylguanine with thymine (5) versus pairing with cytosine (6) may also be understood. Another constraint in respect of steric hindrance also applies and, whilst it is possible to construct a H-bonded base-pair of O^2-methylthymine and guanine, molecular models are excluding, because the O^2-methyl group cannot take up its normal planar configuration on account of the presence of the deoxyribose residue of the nucleotide which is being inserted. Clearly, in situations where the pairing of a template base with incoming nucleotides into the DNA helix conflicts with the highly specific spatial requirement of the active centres of DNA polymerase, this enzyme is inoperative. In contrast, these steric considerations do not apply to RNA polymerase, with which misincorporations appear to occur, even where it is impossible to construct base-pairs.

These concepts are put to the test, for example, by the 3-methylpurines, for which an excision mechanism exists (*see above*), and for which it is possible to draw stable H-bonded base-pairs of either 3-methylguanine (7,8) or 3-methyladenine (9) and the incoming nucleotides (misincorporation would seem to be competitive for the guanine analogue). There is no evidence for the miscoding of 3-methylpurines by DNA polymerase (Abbott and Saffhill, 1977b), however, and steric hindrance may interfere in this molecular situation.

The acceptability of the modified nucleoside 5'-triphosphates, O^6-methyl-dGTP and O^4-methyl-dTTP, as DNA precursors, in an assay *in vitro* using DNA polymerases I and α (Hall and Saffhill, 1983), strongly supports the foregoing suppositions. O^6-Methyl-dGTP was incorporated into the newly synthesized DNA-like material only in the presence of templates containing thymine bases, and O^4-methyl-dTTP was so incorporated only in the presence of templates containing guanine bases (Hall and Saffhill, 1983). Similarly, the fact that the specially prepared poly(dC–3-methyl-dC) does not incur any misincorporation in syntheses of DNA-like material with DNA polymerase I shows that 3-methylcytosine is not promutagenic with regard to DNA polymerases (Saffhill, 1984). These results (Hall and Saffhill, 1983; Saffhill, 1984) confirm the promutagenic nature and base-pairing properties of O^6-methylguanine and O^4-methylthymine.

Again, pertinent cell-culture experiments involving Chinese hamster (V79) cells (Saffhill and Fox, 1980; Brannand, Saffhill and Fox, 1982) showed that out of the O^2-, 3- and O^4-methylthymidines, O^4-methyl-dT was the only nucleoside analogue, which was incorporated into V79 cell DNA, and that addition of thymidine to the cell culture increased the level of O^4-methyl-dT incorporation. The results (Brannand, Saffhill and Fox, 1982) indicated that O^4-methyl-dT is incorporated as an analogue of deoxycytidine into DNA, where it behaves as cytidine during DNA synthesis, in comparison with O^4-methyl-T, which is produced by alkylating carcinogens in somatic DNA, and which is a miscoding promutagenic lesion.

76   Significance of modified deoxyribonucleoside residues in DNA

dC · · · 3-Me-dG   (7)

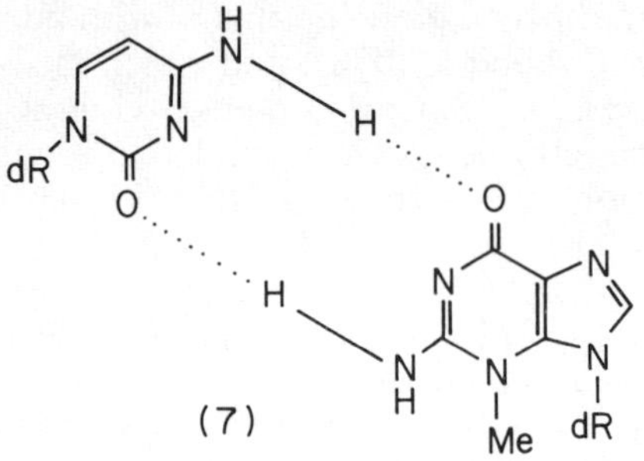

dT · · · 3-Me-dG   (8)

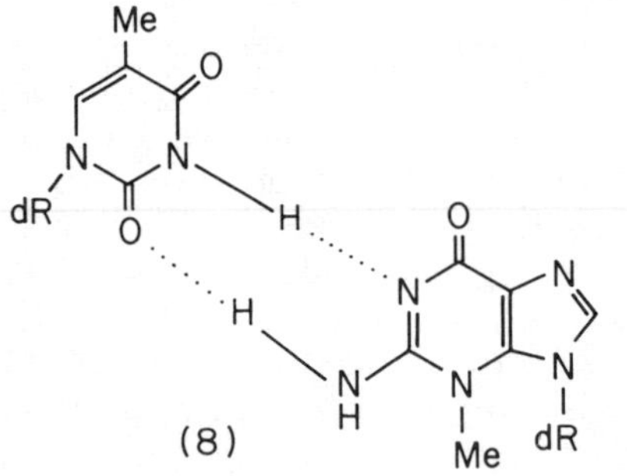

dG · · · 3-Me-dA   (9)

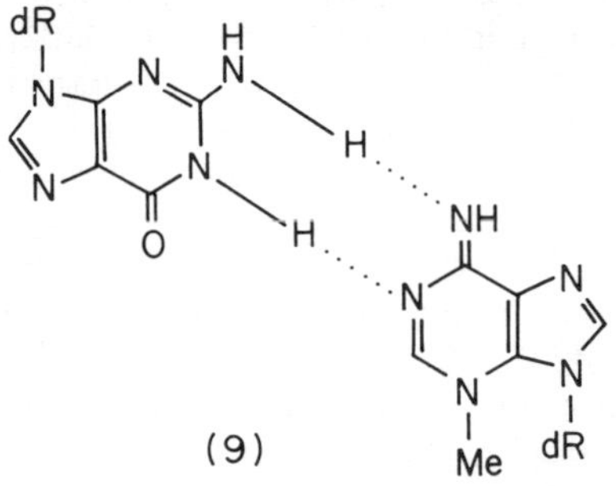

The principal miscodings of O^4-methylthymine, O^4-methyluracil and O^6-methylguanine represent potential promutagenic lesions, which would be expected to lead to (dC–dG) → (dA–dT) transversions, and similarly those of 3-methylpurines may induce (dA–dT) → (dC–dG) transversions. On the foregoing evidence, the predictable induction of these transversions is consistent with the fact that alkylations brought about by N-nitroso compounds induce base-pair-substitution mutations in *Salmonella typhimurium* strains, but not frame-shift mutations (Bartsch, Malaveille and Montesano, 1976). This conclusion (q.v.) agrees with the observation (Coulondre and Miller, 1977) that a large number of (C–G) → (A–T) and a small number of (A–T) → (C–G) transversions result from the action of alkylating agents in bacteria.

In the case of metals which have been shown to be mutagenic or carcinogenic (Flessel, 1979; Langard and Norseth, 1979; IARC, 1980), treatment of the

DNA-like polymer template, poly(dA–dT), with the salts concerned [including Cr^{3+} and Cr^{VI}] led to decreased fidelity with DNA-directed DNA polymerase (Sirover and Loeb, 1976). Chromium(III) is much more potent than Cr^{VI} in causing infidelity of DNA biosynthesis *in vitro* (Sirover and Loeb, 1976). The increased uptake of non-complementary nucleotide (dCTP) incorporated in DNA biosynthesis represents a potential promutagenic lesion that would be expected to lead to (dA–dT) → (dC–dG) transversions. This evidence and reasoning agree with the fact that Cr^{VI} (as chromate or dichromate) is readily taken up by cells but can be easily reduced there to Cr^{3+} by biological reductants (for example, NADPH, ascorbic acid etc.) (Gruber and Jennette, 1978; Petrilla and De Flora, 1978), and that chromium salts induce base-pair-substitution mutations in *Salmonella typhimurium* TA100 strain (IARC, 1980; Stern, 1980). On the other hand, correlation between the alteration in fidelity of DNA biosynthesis *in vitro* and mutagenicity and carcinogenicity *in vivo* agrees with another way of looking at these phenomena, viz. that infidelity during polymerization may cause mutation *per se* (Loeb, Springgate and Battula, 1974; Mitzutani and Temin, 1976).

In the case of the vinyl chloride carcinogen, treatment of DNA-polymer templates, poly(dA–dT) and poly(dC–dG), with vinyl chloride-derived chloroacetaldehyde (Chapters 2, 3) led to deceleration of DNA biosynthesis and decreased fidelity with DNA-directed DNA polymerase (Hall *et al.*, 1981); the *E. coli* DNA polymerase I that was used belongs to the DNA-repair mechanism. With the modified poly(dA–dT) templates, non-complementary dGMP was incorporated to the extent of 1 misincorporation for about every 60 etheno-dA residues (Chapter 3) present, but no misincorporation of non-complementary dCMP occurred, and with the modified poly(dC–dG) templates, 1 misincorporation of either dAMP or dTMP occurred respectively for approximately every 30 or 80 etheno-dC residues (Chapter 3). For the reasons given in Chapter 3, it is reasonable to suppose that formation of ethenoguanine (Oesch and Doerjer, 1982; cf. Kochetov, Shibaev and Kost, 1973) may account for a low proportion (<10%) of the dTMP misincorporations opposite to guanine bases in the modified poly(dC–dG) template (Hall *et al.*, 1981). The principal miscodings of etheno-dA probably represent a potential promutagenic lesion, which would be expected to cause (dA–dT) → (dC–dG) transversions, and etheno-dC would probably induce (dC–dG) → (dA–dT) transversions (Hathway, 1981; *see also*, Barbin *et al.*, 1981; Spengler and Singer, 1981). Hence, induction of (dA–dT) → (dC–dG) and (dC–dG) → (dA–dT) transversions by etheno-dA, etheno-dC and etheno-dG is consistent with the fact that chloroacetaldehyde, chloroethylene oxide and metabolically activated vinyl chloride (Green and Hathway, 1978) induce base-pair-substitution mutations in relevant *Salmonella typhimurium* strains (Rannug *et al.*, 1974; McCann *et al.*, 1975; Malaveille *et al.*, 1975; Phillips, Zahler and Garro, 1980)); vinyl chloride is not a frame-shift mutagen.

The misincorporations envisaged in these biological processes would be facilitated by complex formation involving base-pairing (*Scheme 4.2*). Some of the paired structures involve protonated molecular species, which were invoked to extend the Watson–Crick concept for complementary base-pairing (Topal and Fresco, 1976).

The foregoing evidence confirms results on the kinetics and selectivity of the reaction of chloroacetaldehyde with some tRNA constituents (Biernat *et al.*, 1978), which showed that no nucleoside analogues apart from imidazo-cyclization products were formed.

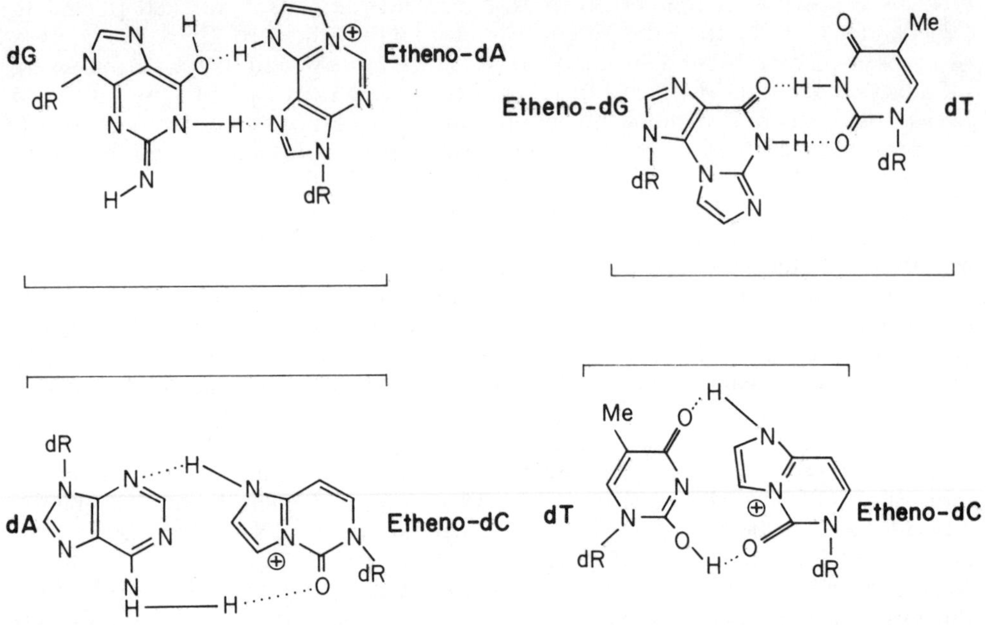

Scheme 4.2

In rather similar work to that with vinyl chloride, aflatoxin B_1 has been reacted with poly(dC–dG), and shown to strongly inhibit DNA-directed DNA polymerase *in vitro* (Chu and Saffhill, 1983). Interpretation of the data for misincorporations was complicated in that at least twice as many apurinic sites were formed as there were aflatoxin residues incorporated. The effect of the apurinic sites was assessed, however, after mild heat depurination which removed all of the 7-substituted aflatoxin B_1–guanine residues. In fact, the aflatoxin residues proved to be stronger inhibitors of DNA polymerases than the apurinic sites are. Apurinic sites induced errors in DNA synthesis *per se*, but up to 280 apurinic sites in poly(dC–dG) were required to cause one misincorporation of dTMP and up to 470 for one misincorporation of dAMP with *E. coli* DNA polymerase I. When appropriate correction was made for these errors, it was found that, for DNA polymerase I, up to 80 aflatoxin B_1-related residues were required for every one misincorporation of a TMP and up to 50 residues for one misincorporation of dAMP (Chu and Saffhill, 1983). Mammalian DNA polymerase α induced errors very similar to the ones found for DNA polymerase I. These values are in fact similar to the estimates calculated by Wogan *et al.* (1979) for the efficiency of the induction of mutations by aflatoxin B_1 adducts in *S. typhimurium* strains and human lymphoblasts. Chu and Saffhill (1983) considered that, whilst the substitution of aflatoxin B_1 residues into the templates produced a strong inhibition of their template function, they did not bring about an absolute blockage to the progression of the enzymes concerned.

Either the misincorporations produced by aflatoxin B_1 occur directly through the copying past a substituent residue, which may have low mutational efficiency or which may be a minor adduct (Wogan *et al.*, 1979), or they may be due to distortions of the DNA helix making the polymers poor, error-prone, templates for the polymerases. A similar pattern of errors was encountered (Barbin *et al.*, 1981;

Hall et al., 1981) for the templates modified by vinyl chloride-related chloroacetaldehyde and also for the ones, modified by N-acetoxy-2AAF (Saffhill and Abbott, 1983).

In that study (Saffhill and Abbott, 1983), N-acetoxy-2AAF reacted with the alternating DNA-like polynucleotides, poly(dC–dG) and poly(dA–dT) *in vitro* to give adducts of guanine and adenine bases similar to those reported in native DNA (Chapter 3). A new guanine residue, formed from N-acetoxy-2AAF, was detected (Saffhill and Abbott, 1983) in the poly(dC–dG), and this was shown not to involve the 7- or 8-positions of guanine. Similarly, a thymine adduct of unknown structure was found in the poly(dA–dT). Modification of the polymers with N-acetoxy-2AAF inhibited their capacity to act as templates for *E. coli* DNA polymerase I and mammalian DNA polymerase α, but the binding of these enzymes to the polynucleotides was unaffected. The modified templates brought about an increase in the levels of misincorporation into newly synthesized DNA.

The point ought to be made that DNA-directed polymerases exemplify biological recognition and enzyme regulation. By emphasizing stability and H-bonded character of the bimolecular complexes that are formed initially in the case of the incoming physiological nucleotides and their analogues (*Schemes 4.1, 4.2*), Saffhill et al. (Saffhill, 1974; Abbott and Saffhill, 1977a,b; Saffhill and Abbott, 1978) have implicitly focused attention on the energy levels of the acceptable complexes, which exclude other prospective substrates that do not form these complexes. Similarly, for example, the dissociation constants of the preferred complexes would be expected to match the corresponding equilibrium constants of the incorporating reactions. Thus, in these enzymically controlled template syntheses, misincorporation occurs only where a nucleotide analogue closely mimics a physiological counterpart and, in this connection, the matter of stable complex formation and the value of its dissociation constant seem to be key factors.

The two foregoing sections of this chapter have been concerned with the direct biological significance of the interactions of reactive carcinogen metabolites with DNA (Chapter 3). Those biochemical lesions which persisted longest in the presence of DNA-repair processes, appeared to be the ones that were most likely to cause miscoding during DNA replication, and investigation of DNA-directed biosynthesis *in vitro* analysed, in fact, the incidence of misincorporations opposite to the various lesions concerned (q.v.). The misincorporations in question lead to transversions, which proved to be the same ones as those detected experimentally in mutagenicity testing (Chapter 2). Hence, some of the initial biochemical lesions (*see above*) correlate strongly with the mutagenicity observed for constituent cells of target tissues. This suggests that chemical carcinogens recognize tissue-sensitive cells, and modify their heritable genetic complement in such a way that another set of genetic events will transform successive generations of these cloned, mutant cells into frank tumours.

Effects on the biosynthesis of inter-related macromolecules

The rest of this chapter deals with alterations in the rate of synthesis of DNA and other cellular macromolecules. Such changes are not envisaged as being concerned specifically with the significance of the foregoing interactions *per se*, but rather they are seen as arising either through the direct interaction of reactive carcinogen metabolites in other biological systems or through the transcription of DNA (which has been modified by carcinogen intervention) with formation of complementary RNA, and through the translation of the genetic message (in the ribosomes) to protein sequencing. Thus, changes in RNA and in protein synthesis would be expected contemporaneous with changes in DNA, and the fact of their occurrence (*see below*) provides strong supporting evidence for the profound changes to somatic DNA economy made by potent carcinogens.

After treatment with DEN, DMN or MNU, protein synthesis in the liver was inhibited, and there was a breakdown of polyribosomes (Magee and Barnes, 1967; Magee and Swann, 1969; Vernie, Bont and Emmelot, 1971; Williams and Hultin, 1973; Stewart, Hicks and Magee, 1975). The mechanism, whereby protein synthesis is inhibited, is incompletely understood, however, but it would appear to involve alkylation since

(*a*) Inhibition of DMN metabolism by aminoacetonitrile prevents this inhibition (Fiume *et al.*, 1970).
(*b*) Simultaneous treatment with cysteamine, which reacts preferentially with the alkylating intermediate generated by DMN (Chapter 2) and reduces significantly the alkylation of cellular macromolecules, prevents this inhibition (Kleihues, Margison and Margison, 1975).
(*c*) The dose–response curve for the inhibition of protein synthesis by DEN and DMN follows the capacity to metabolize these *N*-nitrosamine compounds into alkylating intermediates (Pegg, 1977a).
(*d*) Inhibition is much less clearcut, when the *N*-nitroso compounds were added directly to a protein-synthesizing system *in vitro* (Hradec and Kolar, 1974).

This inhibition of liver-protein synthesis is rather specific since, for example, liver glycolysis and respiration were unaffected (Magee and Barnes, 1967).

It was rational to attribute this inhibition of liver-protein synthesis to a carcinogen-related defect in mRNA (Magee and Barnes, 1967; Pegg, 1977b). Thus alkylation of mRNA (Villa-Trevino, 1967) might make it functionally defective and cause the breakdown of polysomes observed (*see above*). In agreement with this, Pegg and Jackson (1976) found that mRNA was methylated by DMN to a slightly lesser extent than rRNA. It was argued (Magee and Swann, 1969), however, that the resulting small degree of alkylation may have been insufficient to inhibit protein synthesis to the extent observed, as the activity of an alkylated polymer of poly(UG) in a bacterial protein-synthesizing system was decreased by only 40% after 20% of the possible guanosine residues had been alkylated (Wilhelm and Ludlum, 1966), but this reasoning may now need revision. Thus, formation of 7-methylguanine by DMN may bring about an inhibition in mRNA function, even at a low degree of reaction, for the binding to mRNA may occur at sites too far away from initiation sequences to permit translation or to cause premature dissociation of the ribosomes at the time when they would be attempting to translate the sequence containing 7-methylguanosine (Plapp *et al.*, 1974). Nevertheless, the inter-relationship between the synthesis of RNA and that of proteins appears to be complex (Villa-Trevino, 1967; Stewart, Hicks and Magee, 1975).

DMN caused an early lowering in RNA synthesis in the liver (Magee and Barnes, 1967; Villa-Trevino, 1967; Stewart and Magee, 1971; Stewart, Hicks and Magee, 1975; Herzog and Farber, 1976) and kidneys (Stewart and Magee, 1971) of treated rats. Inhibition of RNA synthesis in the kidneys was biphasic with recoveries at days 1 and 5 after treatment, but, after longer treatment, the rate of RNA synthesis both in the liver and in the kidneys may be increased through proliferative regeneration following DMN-induced necrosis (Stewart and Magee, 1971). It appears that the inhibition of hepatic RNA synthesis by DMN may be due to a direct effect on the enzymic activity of RNA polymerase *in vivo* (Herzog and Farber, 1976).

In this connection, Ludlum *et al.* found that formation of 3-ethylcytosine or 3-methylcytosine in a template reaction caused misincorporation of UMP (Ludlum and Wilhelm, 1968; Ludlum, 1970b) with RNA polymerase and that O^6-methylguanine caused misincorporation of UMP and AMP also with RNA polymerase (Gerchman and Ludlum, 1973).

Metal salts, including Cd^{2+} and Pb^{2+} salts, stimulated chain initiation of RNA synthesis at concentrations which inhibited overall RNA synthesis (Hoffman and Niyogi, 1977).

Transcription of calf-thymus DNA that had been modified by reaction with (±)*anti*-BP diol-epoxide with *E. coli* DNA-directed RNA polymerase was increasingly inhibited with increasing incidence of interaction. Inhibition was much greater under conditions which favoured re-initiation of transcription, than under conditions where only one RNA chain was synthesized per initiation site (Leffler *et al.*, 1977). This suggested that the modified sites block the movement of RNA polymerase along the DNA template, and prevent recycling of this enzyme (Leffler *et al.*, 1977).

The inhibition of RNA and protein biosynthesis would be expected to bring about a disturbance in the availability of cellular constituents with a rapid turnover and those marshalled in response to physiological stimuli, for example, α-oxoglutaric acid and glutamic acid in Telodrin convulsive states (Hathway and Mallinson, 1964; Hathway, 1965; Hathway, Mallinson and Akintonwa, 1965).

After treatment with a dose of DMN capable of inducing a 100% incidence of kidney tumours *in vivo*, rat-kidney cells showed, *in vitro*, a marked depression in DNA synthesis which lasted for 1–3 days, and was followed in those cell types that are known to give rise to tumours as opposed to other kidney cells, by increased DNA synthesis and enhanced mitotic activity (Hard, 1975). The time of these increases (Hard, 1975) was in phase with peaks of renal DNA synthesis, at days 3 and 6 after DMN treatment (Stewart and Magee, 1971). Stewart and Magee (1971) also noticed a small peak of thymidine incorporation within 2 hours of DMN administration, which they attributed to repair synthesis. It is relevant that the depression and restoration of DNA synthesis seems to be in phase with a lowering and increase in the activity of cytoplasmic enzymes, including that of DNA polymerase α (Salisbury and O'Connor, 1976; O'Connor, Saffhill and Margison, 1979). Inhibition of DNA synthesis by alkylating agents in cultured mammalian cells is well-known, and the nature of the lesions concerned and their repair has been investigated (Cleaver, 1975; Strauss, Scuderio and Henderson, 1975; Roberts, 1976). It was found (Scuderio and Strauss, 1974) that the growing point of new DNA is delayed by the alkylation lesion and that repair synthesis in the region of the growing point permits continuation of (DNA) synthesis. Thus, a lowering of the rate of DNA synthesis may be due to the time required for gaps, excised in the newly synthesized DNA opposite substituents in the template strand, to be repaired (Roberts, 1976). The time-course for DNA synthesis permits alteration by chemical carcinogen throughout a considerable period of time, and this factor as well as that of the induction and inhibition of enzyme systems both as a result of chemical exposure and of product formation, complicate an interpretation of the mish-mash of observations made with regard to DNA biosynthesis (Saffhill, 1974; Magin *et al.*, 1975; Gol-Winkler and Goutier, 1977).

Finally, it seemed reasonable to include the discussion of the effects on the biosynthesis of inter-related macromolecules in the latter part of this chapter. But, alternatively, discrete parts of this section might have been incorporated, as appropriate, at various stages in the development of Chapter 3, where some of the chemical carcinogens that were mentioned there, particularly the alkylating *N*-nitroso compounds, have been used as experimental tools for tackling problems in relation to macromolecular synthesis. Nevertheless, a continuous discussion of the subject as presently positioned seems to be greatly preferred, since the possibility that the observed effects on the biosynthesis of the inter-related macromolecules reflect carcinogen-modulated changes in the flow of genetic information from DNA to RNA to proteins [Crick's (1970) central dogma of molecular genetics] appears to be incontestible, and accordingly there is a clear relationship between this section and the two preceding ones.

Bibliography and references

ABBOTT, P.J. and SAFFHILL, R. (1977a) *Nucleic Acid Res.*, **4**, 761
ABBOTT, P.J. and SAFFHILL, R. (1977b) *Biochim. Biophys. Acta,* **562**, 51
BARBIN, A., BARTSCH, H., LECONTE, P. and RADMAN, M. (1981) *Nucleic Acid Res.*, **9**, 375
BARTSCH, H., MALAVEILLE, C. and MONTESANO, R. (1976) In *Screening Tests in Chemical Carcinogenesis.* Eds R. Montesano, H. Bartsch and L. Tomatis. International Agency for Research on Cancer Scientific Publications no. 12, pp. 467–486. Lyon, France: IARC
BARTSCH, H., MARGISON, G.P., MALAVEILLE, C., CAMUS, A.M., BRUN, G., MARGISON, J.M. *et al.* (1977) *Arch. Toxikol.*, **39**, 51
BIERANT, J., CIESIOLKA, J., GÓRNICKI, P., ADAMIAK, R.W., KRZYZOSIAK, W.J. and WIEWIOROWSKI, M. (1978) *Nucleic Acid Res.*, **5**, 789
BRANNAND, J., SAFFHILL, R. and FOX, M. (1982) *Carcinogenesis*, **3**, 219
BROOKES, P. and LAWLEY, P.D. (1964) *Nature,* **202**, 781
CAPPS, M.J., O'CONNOR, P.J. and CRAIG, A.W. (1973) *Biochim. Biophys. Acta*, **331**, 33
CHU, Y.-H. and SAFFHILL, R. (1983) *Carcinogenesis*, **4**, 643
CLEAVER, J.E. (1975) *Methods Cancer Res.*, **11**, 123
COOPER, H.K., HAUNENSTEIN, E., KOLAR, G.F. and KLEIHUES, P. (1978) *Acta Neuropathol. (Berlin)*, **43**, 105
COULONDRE, C. and MILLER, J.H. (1977) *J. Mol. Biol.*, **117**, 577
COX, R. and IRVING, C.C. (1977) *Cancer Lett.*, **3**, 265
CRADDOCK, V.M. (1969) *Biochem. J.*, **111**, 497
CRADDOCK, V.M. (1975a) *Chem.-Biol. Interact.*, **10**, 313
CRADDOCK, V.M. (1975b) *Chem.-Biol. Interact.*, **10**, 323
CRICK, F.H.C. (1970) *Nature,* **227**, 516
DE MUNTER, H.K., DEN ENGELSE, L. and EMMELOT, P. (1979) *Chem.-Biol. Interact.*, **24**, 299
DEN ENGELSE, L. (1974) *Chem.-Biol. Interact.*, **8**, 329
DRUCKREY, H. and KÜPFMÜLLER, K. (1948) *Z. Naturforschung,* **3B**, 254
DRUCKREY, H. and KÜPFMÜLLER, K. (1949) *Dosis und Wirkung.* Aulendorf-im-Württemberg: Editio Cantor
DRUCKREY, H., PREUSSMAN, R., IVANKOVIC, S. and SCHMÄHL, D. (1967) *Z. Krebsforschung*, **69**, 103
FIUME, L., CAMPADELLI-FIUME, G., MAGEE, P.N. and HOLSMAN, J. (1970) *Biochem. J.*, **120**, 601
FLESSEL, C.P. (1979) *Trace Metals in Health and Disease.* pp. 109–122. New York: Raven Press
FRAVALL, H.N.A. and ROBERTS, J.J. (1978) *Chem.-Biol. Interact.*, **23**, 99
FREI, J.V. and LAWLEY, P.D. (1975) *Chem.-Biol. Interact.*, **10**, 413
FREI, J.V., SWENSON, D.H., WARREN, W. and LAWLEY, P.D. (1978) *Biochem. J.*, **174**, 1031
GERCHMAN, L.L. and LUDLUM, D.B. (1973) *Biochim. Biophys. Acta,* **308**, 310
GOL-WINKLER, R. and GOUTIER, R. (1977) *Eur. J. Cancer,* **13**, 1081
GOTH, R. and RAJEWSKY, M.F. (1972) *Cancer Res.*, **32**, 1501
GOTH, R. and RAJEWSKY, M.F. (1974a) *Z. Krebsforschung*, **82**, 37
GOTH, R. and RAJEWSKY, M.F. (1974b) *Proc. Natl Acad. Sci. USA*, **71**, 639

GREEN, T. and HATHWAY, D.E. (1978) *Chem.-Biol. Interact.*, **22**, 211
GRUBER, J.E. and JENNETTE, K.W. (1978) *Biochem. Biophys. Res. Commun.*, **82**, 700
HALL, J.A. and SAFFHILL, R. (1983) *Nucleic Acid Res.*, **11**, 4185
HALL, J.A., SAFFHILL, R., GREEN, T. and HATHWAY, D.E. (1981) *Carcinogenesis*, **2**, 141
HARD, G.C. (1975) *Cancer Res.*, **35**, 3762
HATHWAY, D.E. (1965) *Arch. Environ. Hlth*, **11**, 380
HATHWAY, D.E. (1981) *Br. J. Cancer*, **44**, 597
HATHWAY, D.E. and MALLINSON, A. (1964) *Biochem. J.*, **90**, 51
HATHWAY, D.E., MALLINSON, A. and AKINTONWA, D.A.A. (1965) *Biochem. J.*, **94**, 676
HERZOG, J. and FARBER, J.L. (1976) *Cancer Res.*, **36**, 1761
HOFFMAN, D.J. and NIYOGI, S.K. (1977) *Science*, **198**, 513
HRADEC, J. and KOLAR, G.F. (1974) *Chem.-Biol. Interact.*, **8**, 243
INTERNATIONAL AGENCY FOR RESEARCH ON CANCER (1980) *Monographs on the Risk of Chemicals to Humans: Some Metals and Metallic Compounds.* Vol. 23, pp. 205–323. Lyon, France: IARC
JONES, H.B. and GRENDON, A. (1975) *Food Cosmet. Toxicol.*, **13**, 251
KIRTIKAR, D.M., DIPPLE, A. and GOLDTHWAIT, D.A. (1975) *Biochemistry*, **14**, 5548
KIRTIKAR, D.M. and GOLDTHWAIT, D.A. (1974) *Proc. Natl Acad. Sci. USA*, **71**, 2022
KLEIHUES, P. and BÜCHELER, J. (1977) *Nature*, **269**, 625
KLEIHUES, P. and MAGEE, P.N. (1973) *J. Neurochem.*, **20**, 595
KLEIHUES, P. and MARGISON, G.P. (1974) *J. Natl Cancer Inst.*, **53**, 1839
KLEIHUES, P. and MARGISON, G.P. (1976) *Nature*, **259**, 153
KLEIHUES, P., MARGISON, J.M. and MARGISON, G.P. (1975) *Cancer Res.*, **35**, 3667
KOCHETOV, N.K., SHIBAEV, V.N. and KOST, A.A. (1973) *Dokl. Akad. Nauk SSSR*, **213**, 1327
KRIEG, D.R. (1963) *Genetics*, **48**, 561
LANGARD, S. and NORSETH, T. (1979) In *Handbook on the Toxicology of Metals.* Ed L. Friberg. pp. 383–397. Amsterdam: Elsevier/North Holland Biomedical Press
LAWLEY, P.D. (1966) *Prog. Nucleic Acid Res. Mol. Biol.*, **5**, 89
LAWLEY, P.D. (1976) In *Screening Tests in Chemical Carcinogenesis*. Eds R. Montesano, H. Bartsch and L. Tomatis. IARC Scientific Publications, no. 12, pp. 181–208. Lyon, France: IARC
LAWLEY, P.D. and BROOKES, P. (1961) *Nature*, **192**, 1081
LAWLEY, P.D. and ORR, D.J. (1970) *Chem.-Biol. Interact.*, **2**, 154
LAWLEY, P.D., ORR, D.J. and SHAH, S.A. (1971/1972) *Chem.-Biol. Interact.*, **4**, 431
LAWLEY, P.D., ORR, D.J., SHAH, S.A., FARMER, P.B. and JARMAN, M. (1973) *Biochem. J.*, **135**, 193
LEFFLER, S., PULKABECK, P., GRUNBERGER, D. and WEINSTEIN, I.B. (1977) *Biochemistry*, **16**, 3133
LIEBERMAN, M.W. and DIPPLE, A. (1972) *Cancer Res.*, **32**, 1855
LIKHACHEV, A.J., MARGISON, G.P. and MONTESANO, R. (1977) *Chem.-Biol. Interact.*, **18**, 235
LOEB, L.A., SPRINGGATE, C.F. and BATTULA, N. (1974) *Cancer Res.*, **34**, 2311
LOEB, L.A., WEYMOUTH, L.A., KUNKEL, T.A., GOPINATHAN, K.P., BECKMAN, R.A. and DUKE, D.K. (1980) *Cold Spring Harb. Symp. Quant. Biol.*, **43**
LOVELESS, A. (1969) *Nature*, **223**, 206
LUDLUM, D.B. (1970a) *J. Biol. Chem.*, **245**, 477
LUDLUM, D.B. (1970b) *Biochim. Biophys. Acta*, **213**, 142
LUDLUM, D.B. and WILHELM, R.C. (1968) *J. Biol. Chem.*, **243**, 2750
McCANN, J., SIMMON, V., STREITWIESER, D. and AMES, B.N. (1975) *Proc. Natl Acad. Sci. USA*, **73**, 3190
McELHONE, M.J., O'CONNOR, P.J. and CRAIG, A.W. (1971) *Biochem. J.*, **125**, 821
MAGEE, P.N. and BARNES, J.M. (1967) *Adv. Cancer Res.*, **10**, 163
MAGEE, P.N. and SWANN, P.F. (1969) *Br. Med. Bull.*, **25**, 240
MAGIN, M.N., O'CONNOR, P.J., CRAIG, A.W. and MARGISON, G.P. (1975) *Z. Krebsforschung*, **84**, 217
MALAVEILLE, C., BARTSCH, H., BARBIN, A., CAMUS, A.M. and MONTESANO, R. (1975) *Biochem. Biophys. Res. Commun.*, **63**, 363
MARGISON, G.P. and KLEIHUES, P. (1975) *Biochem. J.*, **148**, 521
MARGISON, G.P. and O'CONNOR, P.J. (1973) *Biochim. Biophys. Acta*, **331**, 349
MARGISON, G.P., CAPPS, M.J., O'CONNOR, P.J. and CRAIG, A.W. (1973) *Chem.-Biol. Interact.*, **6**, 119
MARGISON, G.P., LIKHACHEV, A.J. and KOLAR, G.F. (1979) *Chem.-Biol. Interact.*, **25**, 345
MARGISON, G.P., MARGISON, J.M. and MONTESANO, R. (1976) *Biochem. J.*, **157**, 627
MARGISON, G.P., MARGISON, J.M. and MONTESANO, R. (1977) *Biochem. J.*, **165**, 463
MARGISON, G.P., MARGISON, J.M. and MONTESANO, R. (1979) *Biochem. J.*, **177**, 967
MARGISON, G.P. and O'CONNOR, P.J. (1979) In *Chemical Carcinogens and DNA.* Ed. P.L. Grover. Vol. 1, pp. 111–159. Boca Raton, Florida: CRC Press
MITZUTANI, S. and TEMIN, H.M. (1976) *Biochemistry*, **15**, 1510
NICOLL, J.W., SWANN, P.F. and PEGG, A.E. (1975) *Nature*, **254**, 261

NICOLL, J.W., SWANN, P.F. and PEGG, A.E. (1977) *Chem.-Biol. Interact.*, **16**, 301
O'CONNOR, P.J., CAPPS, M.J. and CRAIG, A.W. (1973) *Br. J. Cancer*, **27**, 153
O'CONNOR, P.J., SAFFHILL, R. and MARGISON, G.P. (1979) In *Environmental Carcinogenesis*. Eds P. Emmelot and E. Kriek. pp. 73–96. Amsterdam: Elsevier/North Holland Biomedical Press
OESCH, F. and DOERJER, G. (1982) *Carcinogenesis*, **3**, 663
PEGG, A.E. (1977a) *J. Natl Cancer Inst.*, **58**, 681
PEGG, A.E. (1977b) *Adv. Cancer Res.*, **25**, 195
PEGG, A.E. (1978a) *Chem.-Biol. Interact.*, **22**, 109
PEGG, A.E. (1978b) *Biochem. Biophys. Res. Commun.*, **84**, 166
PEGG, A.E. and HUI, G. (1978a) *Cancer Res.*, **38**, 2011
PEGG, A.E. and HUI, G. (1978b) *Biochem. J.*, **173**, 739
PEGG, A.E. and JACKSON, A. (1976) *Chem.-Biol. Interact.*, **12**, 279
PEGG, A.E. and NICOLL, J.W. (1976) In *Screening Tests in Chemical Carcinogenesis*. Eds R. Montesano, H. Bartsch and L. Tomatis. IARC Scientific Publications, no. 12, pp. 571–592. Lyon, France: IARC
PETRILLA, F.L. and DE FLORA, S. (1978) *Mutat. Res.*, **54**, 139
PHILLIPS, D.H., GROVER, P.L. and SIMS, P. (1978) *Int. J. Cancer*, **22**, 487
PHILLIPS, R.A., ZAHLER, S.A. and GARRO, A.J. (1980) *Mutat. Res.*, **74**, 267
PLAPP, F.V., HAYES, L.C., TILZER, L. and CHIGA, M. (1974) *Nature*, **247**, 311
RANNUG, U., JOHANSSON, A., RAMEL, C. and WACHTMEISTER, C.A. (1974) *Ambio*, **3**, 194
RAYMAN, M.P. and DIPPLE, A. (1973) *Biochemistry*, **12**, 1538
REGAN, J.D. and SETLOW, R.B. (1974) *Cancer Res.*, **34**, 3318
ROBERTS, J.J. (1976) In *Screening Tests in Chemical Carcinogenesis*. Eds R. Montesano, H. Bartsch and L. Tomatis. IARC Scientific Publications, no. 12, pp. 605–612. Lyon, France: IARC
ROBERTS, J.J. and THOMSON, A.J. (1979) *Prog. Nucleic Acid. Res. Mol. Biol.*, **22**, 71
ROBERTS, J.J. and WARD, K.N. (1973) *Chem.-Biol. Interact.*, **7**, 241
SAFFHILL, R. (1974) *Biochem. Biophys. Res. Commun.*, **61**, 802
SAFFHILL, R. (1984) *Carcinogenesis*, **5**, In the press
SAFFHILL, R. and ABBOTT, P.J. (1978) *Nucleic Acid Res.*, **5**, 1971
SAFFHILL, R. and ABBOTT, P.J. (1983) *Chem.-Biol. Interact.*, **44**, 95
SAFFHILL, R. and FOX, M. (1980) *Carcinogenesis*, **1**, 487
SALISBURY, J.G. and O'CONNOR, P.J. (1976) *Nucleic Acid Res.*, **3**, 1561
SCHOENTAL, R. (1967) *Biochem. J.*, **102**, 5C
SCUDIERO, D. and STRAUSS, B. (1974) *J. Mol. Biol.*, **83**, 17
SINGER, B. (1976) *Nature*, **264**, 333
SINGER, B. and FRAENKEL-CONRAT, H. (1970) *Biochemistry*, **9**, 3694
SINGER, B., FRAENKEL-CONRAT, H. and KUŚMIEREK, J.T. (1978) *Proc. Natl Acad. Sci. USA*, **75**, 1722
SIROVER, M.A. and LOEB, L.A. (1976) *Science*, **194**, 1434
SPENGLER, S. and SINGER, B. (1981) *Nucleic Acid Res.*, **9**, 365
STERN, R.M. (1980) *A Chemical, Physical and Mutagenic Assay of Welding Fumes*. Proceedings of the First International Workshop in *in vitro* Effects of Fibrous Dust, MRC Pneumoconiosis Research Unit, Cardiff (1979). London: Academic Press
STEWART, B.W. and MAGEE, P.N. (1971) *Biochem. J.*, **125**, 943
STEWART, B.W., HICKS, R.M. and MAGEE, P.N. (1975) *Chem.-Biol. Interact.*, **11**, 413
STRAUSS, B., SCUDIERO, D. and HENDERSON, E. (1975) In *Molecular Mechanisms for the Repair of DNA*. Eds P. Hanawalt and R. Setlow. pp. 13–24. New York: Plenum Press
STUMPF, R., MARGISON, G.P., MONTESANO, R. and PEGG, A.E. (1979) *Cancer Res.*, **39**, 50
SWANN, P.F. and MAGEE, P.N. (1968) *Biochem. J.*, **110**, 39
SWANN, P.F. and MAGEE, P.N. (1971) *Biochem. J.*, **125**, 841
SWENBERG, J.A., COOPER, H.K., BÜCHELER, J. and KLEIHUES, P. (1979) *Cancer Res.*, **39**, 465
TERRACINI, B., MAGEE, P.N. and BARNES, J.M. (1967) *Br. J. Cancer*, **21**, 559
TOPAL, M.D. and FRESCO, J.R. (1976) *Nature*, **263**, 285
VAN DEN BERG, H.W. and ROBERTS, J.J. (1975a) *Chem.-Biol. Interact.*, **11**, 493
VAN DEN BERG, H.W. and ROBERTS, J.J. (1975b) *Mutat. Res.*, **33**, 279
VERNIE, L.N., BONT, W.S. and EMMELOT, P. (1971) *Cancer Res.*, **31**, 2189
VILLA-TREVINO, S. (1967) *Biochem. J.*, **105**, 625
WILHELM, R.C. and LUDLUM, D.B. (1966) *Science*, **153**, 1403
WILLIAMS, G.M. and HULTIN, T. (1973) *Cancer Res.*, **33**, 1796
WOGAN, G.N., CORY, R.G., ESSIGMANN, J.M., GROOPMAN, J.D., THILLY, W.G., SKOPEK, T.R. *et al.* (1979) In *Environmental Carcinogenesis, Risk Evaluation and Mechanisms*. Eds P. Emmelot and E. Kriek. pp. 97–121. Amsterdam: Elsevier

Chapter 5

Mechanisms in perspectives: inhibition of tumour induction

An unfolding scientific literature discloses the results of investigations relating to the inhibition of chemical carcinogenesis by means of various agents, including hindered phenolic antioxidants, and these observations now enable an attempt to be made to rationalize this field.

The foregoing ideas infer that work on the inhibition of tumour induction by chemical carcinogens (*see below*) may be interpreted in terms of the mechanisms which have been proposed (*see* Chapters 2–4). This suggests, by corollary, that a survey of the inhibitory effects would put the causative mechanism of chemical carcinogenesis (q.v.) into perspective. From the point of view of industrial hygiene on the other hand, the possibility of introducing prophylaxis is not very attractive in circumstances relating to the manufacture of a frank carcinogen in a specially designed chemical plant from which there is very little risk of exposure. Moreover, the use of such preventive measures may not be entirely effective in the case of an accidental overwhelming exposure. The concept that such investigations might lead to the raising of apparent thresholds for specific industrial chemicals is more interesting, however, and such a proposition might be valuable in certain circumstances to a committed governmental agency.

The idea of inhibitors and promoters of tumour induction derives historically from Berenblum's discovery (1929) of 2,2'-dichlorodiethyl sulphide as a potent 'anti-carcinogen' for mouse skin and of crude croton resin as a 'co-carcinogen' for mouse skin pre-treated with benzo[α]pyrene (Berenblum, 1941; *see also* Berenblum, 1974). It follows theoretically that it ought to be possible to raise or lower the potency of prospective mutagens/carcinogens, and this seems to be so, as hindered phenolic antioxidants, such as BHA (a mixture of 2- and 3-*tert*-butyl-4-methoxyphenol) and BHT (3,5-di-*tert*-butyl-4-hydroxytoluene), reduce the potential of a chemical carcinogen to cause chromosome breaks (Shamberger *et al.*, 1973) and to induce tumours (Wattenberg, 1973).

The present chapter emphasizes that inhibitory effects to tumour induction may occur:

(*a*) Before DNA injury by amongst other things:
    (i) The inhibition of enzyme system(s) responsible for metabolic activation of the carcinogen.
    (ii) The induction of the detoxifying disposition of reactive carcinogen intermediates.

(iii) The provision of a source of exogenous nucleophiles (*see above*).
(*b*) After modification of target-organ DNA, by:
(i) Affecting excision–repair or postreplication repair.

Clearly, in some cases, the operation of more than one mechanism may be involved. In addition, a caveat ought to be entered to the effect that the empirical discovery of inhibitory effects sometimes outstrips a fitting explanation. Finally, this chapter is properly located, as the subject matter relates to that of the preceding ones.

Inhibition of tumour initiation by metabolic inducers and inhibitors

Treatment of rats with 2,6-dichloro-4-nitrophenol or pentachlorophenol 45 min before administration of *N*-(2-fluorenyl)acetamide (2AAF) completely inhibited the hepatotoxic effects of 2AAF in those animals (Meerman and Mulder, 1981). 2,6-Dichloro-4-nitrophenol and pentachlorophenol are known inhibitors of the N–O sulphation, which represents the second stage in the metabolic activation of 2AAF. Prevention of esterification, and thus of full activation, mitigates against DNA injury.

Phenobarbital and polychlorinated biphenyls (the Aroclors) are well-established inducers of mixed function oxidases, and it is an interesting exercise to unravel their sometimes complex actions with regard to the tumorigenicity of notable chemical carcinogens. Thus, in rats which had been chronically pre-treated with phenobarbital, the carcinogenicity of 2AAF was diminished (Wyatt and Cramer, 1970; Peraino, Fry and Staffeldt, 1971), and the chronic pre-treatment with phenobarbital was found (Matsushima *et al.*, 1972) predictably to increase excretion of hydroxylated 2AAF metabolites including the *N*-hydroxy compound. Furthermore, the amount of carcinogen-derived label that was bound to liver DNA was only about one-half of that in the positive control animals (Matsushima *et al.*, 1972), and these authors found a greatly increased excretion of glucuronides, particularly of that of *N*-hydroxy-*N*-(2-fluorenyl)acetamide (*see also* Weisburger and Weisburger, 1973). We now know that phenobarbital induces UDP-glucuronyl transferase activity.

On the other hand, phenobarbital, in its role as an inducer of cytochrome P450, increased 2AAF carcinogenicity (Peraino, Fry and Staffeldt, 1971), when it was administered to rats after the carcinogen (Peraino *et al.*, 1980).

In a rather similar way, pre-treatment of animals with phenobarbital diminished DEN carcinogenicity (Peraino *et al.*, 1973). It appears that phenobarbital accelerated the cytochrome P450 metabolic activation of DEN but also increased, to a greater extent, the activity of *S*-glutathione transferase, which assists the removal of the Me-N$_2^+$ cations produced.

The same sort of picture emerged from investigations where rats were given a carcinogenic diet containing 2AAF and supplemented with the hindered phenolic antioxidant, BHT (Goodman, Trosko and Yager, 1976). In contrast to the control animals, which did not receive BHT, the BHT-treated animals continued to grow and the incidence of tumours in them was small compared with that in the controls (Goodman, Trosko and Yager, 1976). Parallel feeding experiments (Ulland *et al.*, 1972; Grantham, Weisburger and Weisburger, 1973) showed that much larger amounts of the *N*-hydroxy derivative of 2AAF was excreted as glucuronide more rapidly in animals, where the carcinogen had been supplemented with BHT. Hence, it was suspected that the inhibition by BHT of 2AAF tumours was due to the metabolic induction of the enzymes concerned with the detoxifying disposition of the reactive N-hydroxy-2AAF metabolite. This appears to be the case, as BHA produced marked increases in cytoplasmic UDP-glucose dehydrogenase and microsomal UDP-glucuronyl transferase in the livers of CD-1 mice *in vivo*, which implied a greatly increased capacity for synthesis of glucuronide metabolites (Cha and Bueding, 1979; Talalay *et al.*, 1979). Studies involving cell culture showed that BHT had no effect either on excision–repair or on postreplication repair of DNA (Goodman, Trosko and Yager, 1976). The parallel animal-feeding experiments (Goodman, Trosko and Yager, 1976) indicated that the inhibitory effect of BHT was exerted prior to the initiation of DNA injury.

In their investigations of benzo[α]pyrene metabolism by mouse-liver microsomes both from normal animals and from ones fed BHA, Lam and Wattenberg (1977) accounted for the inhibitory effect of BHA on benzo[α]pyrene-induced carcinogenesis in terms of (*a*) the greatly increased induction of aromatic hydroxylation in the 3-position and the detoxifying disposition of carcinogen thereby, and (*b*) a significant decrease in effective epoxidation (the activation process for benzo[α]pyrene carcinogenesis). Other work (Talalay *et al.*, 1979) showed that BHA greatly diminished the production of mutagenic urine in animals exposed to benzo[α]pyrene, and that the antioxidant vastly induced epoxide hydratase and *S*-glutathione transferase activities, which would facilitate rapid detoxication of the reactive carcinogen metabolite(s).

This interpretation of the inhibition of benzo[α]pyrene carcinogenicity by hindered phenolic antioxidants is supported by complementary work on another polycyclic aromatic hydrocarbon. Thus, Slaga and Bracken (1977) established that BHA and BHT, as well as vitamins C and E, inhibit the induction of 7,12-dimethylbenz[α]anthracene tumours in mouse skin. These antioxidants did not significantly induce aryl hydroxylation, but when either BHA or BHT was applied topically to mice, the epidermally mediated covalent binding of 7,12-dimethylbenz[α]anthracene or benzo[α]pyrene material to DNA was inhibited *in vitro*. Addition of either BHA or BHT *in vitro*, however, did not inhibit the epidermally mediated covalent binding of polycyclic aromatic hydrocarbon metabolites to DNA (Slaga and Bracken, 1977). These results apparently exclude the direct interaction of antioxidant and reactive carcinogen metabolite, but relate inhibition of tumorigenesis to the capacity of these antioxidants to either (*a*) inhibit metabolic activation of polycyclic aromatic hydrocarbons via their epoxide derivatives *in vivo*, or (*b*) induce the detoxifying disposition of the reactive intermediates in the intact cells (Berry *et al.*, 1977; Slaga and Bracken, 1977) in the way which has been described by Talalay *et al.* (1979).

If the foregoing explanation of skin-cancer inhibition by antioxidants is correct then, predictably, it ought to be possible to increase say benzo[α]pyrene carcinogenesis by the administration of an epoxide-hydratase inhibitor. That this seems to be the case was shown by Karamysheva, Koblyakov and Turusov (1980), who found that the co-administration of carcinogen and 1,1,1-trichloro-2-propene oxide to mice increased both the rate of appearance of tumours and their incidence compared with that found in positive control animals. Stimulation of benzo[α]pyrene- and of 3-methylcholanthrene-induced mouse-skin cancer by 1,1,1-trichloro-2-propene oxide (Karamysheva, Koblyakov and Turusov, 1980) is due to the capacity of this substance to inhibit epoxide hydratase and to reduce the level of intracellular glutathione, and to the resulting increase in concentration of the reactive carcinogen intermediates.

On the other hand, the retardation of 7,12-dimethylbenz[α]anthracene-induced buccal pouch carcinogenesis in hamsters by 1,4-dimethylnaphthalene and phenanthrene (Malament and Shklar, 1981) appears to be an interesting case of analogue blockade. Enzyme induction/inhibition is not involved.

Busk and Ahborg (1980) found that retinol inhibited aflatoxin B_1 mutagenicity in the Ames *Salmonella typhimurium*/mammalian microsome assay (Chapter 2) and the inhibitory effect was dose dependent, but the mutagenicity of the direct-acting carcinogen, 1,2,3,4-diepoxybutane, was unaffected by retinol. Clearly, the vitamin does not provide a source of nucleophiles for reactive carcinogen epoxides, but inhibition of the mutagen, aflatoxin B_1-2,3-epoxide, depends on the greatly enhanced epoxide hydratase and *S*-glutathione transferase activities induced by antioxidants, retinoids etc. (Talalay *et al.*, 1979).

Benzyl, phenyl and phenethyl isothiocyanates (R−N=C=S) inhibited 7,12-dimethylbenz[α]anthracene-induced mammary tumour formation in female Sprague–Dawley rats, when given 4 h before the carcinogen, but not when administered 24 h before or 4 h after carcinogen (Wattenberg, 1977). Addition of either of the naturally occurring isothiocyanates, benzyl or phenethyl isothiocyanates, to a diet containing 7,12-dimethylbenz[α]anthracene inhibited the induction of tumours of the forestomach and pulmonary adenomas in female ICR/Ha mice. A benzo[α]pyrene-containing diet supplemented with benzyl isothiocyanate also inhibited carcinogenesis of the mouse forestomach (Wattenberg, 1977). Limited information available suggests that organic isothiocyanates induce the detoxifying disposition of reactive carcinogen epoxides. The two anutrient plant metabolites, benzyl and phenethyl isothiocyanates, which occur in Brussels sprouts, cabbage, cauliflower, kale, turnips and watercress (*Cruciferae*), inhibit chemical carcinogenesis and, thus, lower the apparent exposure resulting from chemical carcinogens in carcinogenicity testing.

When sodium cyanate was added to the diet of female Sprague–Dawley rats 8 days before they were challenged with 7,12-dimethylbenz[α]anthracene, it inhibited 7,12-dimethylbenz[α]anthracene-induced mammary neoplasia and, in the diet of ICR/Ha mice, it inhibited benzo[α]pyrene-induced tumours of the forestomach and lungs (Wattenberg, 1980). There are some similarities between the chemical properties of OCN^- and the organic isothiocyanates but, on existing evidence, the mechanism by which OCN^- inhibits polycyclic aromatic hydrocarbon carcinogenesis cannot be deduced.

Treatment of CDF rats exposed to 1,2-dimethylhydrazine with disulphiram (1) caused increased pulmonary excretion of azomethane, diminished production of carcinogen-derived CO_2, and decreased elimination of unchanged 1,2-dimethylhydrazine in the urine (Fiala *et al.*, 1977). Both compound (1) and its

$$Et_2NCS-SCNEt_2$$
$$\parallel \quad \parallel$$
$$S \quad S$$

(1)

↓

$$Et_2NCSH$$
$$\parallel$$
$$S$$

(2)

N,N-diethyldithiocarbamate metabolite (2) inhibit the activity of cytochrome P450 and cytochrome P420 enzyme systems (Lang, Marselos and Törrönen, 1976; Zemaitis and Greene, 1976), and this would account for the diminished output of carcinogen-derived CO_2 in the investigation (Fiala et al., 1977). The induction of the conversion of 1,2-dimethylhydrazine into azomethane by disulphiram is independent of cytochromes P450 and P420 and of the production of the methylating Me-N_2^+ cations (Chapter 2). This interpretation of these data (Fiala et al., 1977) explains Wattenberg's finding (1975) that compound (1) completely prevented 1,2-dimethylhydrazine-induced tumorigenesis of the large intestine (in rats).

Two decades ago, it had been found (Druckrey et al., 1964) that N-n-butyl-N-(4-hydroxybutyl)nitrosamine (BHBN) caused urinary bladder cancer in rats, and a recent investigation (Irving, Tice and Murphy, 1979) has established that compound (1) inhibited significantly such induction of cancer. It is fair comment that the mechanism by which compound (1) inhibits the induction of BHBN bladder cancer has not yet been properly established, but it is likely to impinge on BHBN metabolism in vivo. Thus, compound (1) is a well-known inhibitor of the aldehyde dehydrogenases (Dietrich and Erwin, 1971), and probably inhibits the oxidation of BHBN into its major metabolite, N-n-butyl-N-(3-carboxypropyl)nitrosamine (BCPN), which is postulated (Okado, 1976; Okado and Ishidate, 1977) to be a BHBN proximate carcinogenic metabolite. In support of this possibility, (a) the pre-treatment of rats with α-naphthylisothiocyanate significantly decreased the induction of BHBN bladder tumours (Ito et al., 1974), and (b) 13-cis-retinoic acid also diminished the number and severity of bladder tumours induced by BHBN in rats (Grubbs et al., 1977) and mice (Becci et al., 1978). Disulphiram is a known inducer of glucuronyl transferase (Marselos, Lang and Törrönen, 1976), and it probably acts in this way as well in the work of Irving, Tice and Murphy (1979) which has been described, thereby accelerating the detoxifying disposition of BCPN. Similarly, in the work of Ito et al. (1974) as well, α-naphthylisothiocyanate would seem to induce glucuronyl transferase. Accordingly, there is pretty good evidence for inhibition of the major oxidative step in the causative mechanism of BHBN, and for accelerated removal of a major proximate metabolite (BCPN), which together would appear to account for the inhibition of the BHBN bladder cancer observed (Irving, Tice and Murphy, 1979).

Predictably, since compound (1) is an inhibitor of cytochrome P450 and P420 (Lang, Marselos and Törrönen, 1976; Zemaitis and Greene, 1976), it would be expected to inhibit the tumour-initiating capacity of animals exposed to carcinogenic polycyclic aromatic hydrocarbons by inhibiting mediated epoxidations. Wattenberg's findings (1974) show that, in fact, compound (1) inhibited benzo[a]pyrene-induced tumours of the forestomach in mice and 7,12-dimethylbenz[a]anthracene-induced mammary tumours in female rats.

Complication may arise in respect of the direct-acting intragastric stomach and small intestine carcinogens, N-methyl-N'-nitro-N-nitrosoguanidine (MNNG) and N-methyl-N-nitrosourea (MNU). They do not require enzyme-catalysed reactions to form electrophiles (Schultz and McCalla, 1969; Lawley and Thatcher, 1970; So, Magadia and Wynder, 1973; Wattenberg, 1974), and any metabolism of them can result only in detoxication. Thus, in the case of animals treated with MNNG or MNU, the administration of a metabolic inhibitor, for example disulphiram, would actually potentiate the tumorigenic effects. In some cases of tumour inhibition, where an interpretation is complicated, the biological events immediately after dosing are cardinal to the initiation of a tumorigenic response especially where, for example, a single intrarectal administration of MNNG actually causes tumour induction in the colon (Narisawa et al., 1976).

Interestingly, a protein-deficient diet, which decreases microsomal activity (Czygan et al., 1974) would by the same token potentiate MNNG mutagenicity/carcinogenicity (Popper et al., 1973). Similar interference with the enzymic disposition of the direct-acting nitrogen mustards would also potentiate their tumorigenic effects.

The use of substances which are capable of inducing and/or inhibiting enzyme activities, with carcinogens which potentially affect several tissues, can lead to a shift in overt target organ. Thus, for example, disulphiram which inhibits the metabolic activation of DEN and DMN and which abolishes the corresponding incidence of liver tumours, increases the incidence of oesophageal tumours in proportion to the decrease in liver-tumour incidence (Schmähl et al., 1976). Presumably, the small proportion of a dose of DEN and DMN, which is normally taken-up near the site of (oral) administration by the oesophageal epithelium, is metabolically activated in quantity incommensurate with the expression of mutagenicity. But, where the hepatic metabolism of DEN or DMN is inhibited or blocked, for example by disulphiram, a consequent change in the distribution of unmetabolized N-nitroso compound makes larger amounts available to the oesophagus, where tumours are eventually formed. In respect of DEN and DMN carcinogenesis, therefore, disulphiram confers no benefit whatever to the animals exposed.

In other researches, Narisawa et al. (1976) found that rats fed a retinol-deficient diet had an increased incidence of tumours of the urinary bladder but a diminished incidence of colon tumours after intrarectal administration of MNNG, compared with MNNG-treated rats fed standard diet or a retinol-supplemented diet. On the other hand, rats given a diet supplemented with retinol had fewer adenocarcinomas of the colon after intrarectal MNNG than MNNG-treated rats on a standard diet (Narisawa et al., 1976). These two sets of results are apparently anomalous, but it must be remembered that MNNG is a direct-acting carcinogen. In the first experiments, retinol deficiency makes the bladder epithelium more susceptible to tumour induction than that of the colon, and more MNNG is utilized in initiating bladder cancer at the expense of the colon, where in consequence a lower incidence of tumours results. In the second experiments, where the animals had been equilibrated with retinol, the vitamin accelerated the detoxifying disposition of an intrarectal dose of MNNG, with the result that the amount taken-up by the colon epithelium was commensurate with fewer tumours than in the control animals, and that taken-up by the bladder epithelium was incommensurate with the induction of bladder tumours, whereas, in those animals on a standard diet containing MNNG, the distribution of carcinogen is consistent with the induction of colon adenocarcinomas and of some bladder tumours. Cancer prevention by retinoids seems to be promising (Meyskens and Prasad, 1983).

A special case of the inhibition of tumour induction is instanced by riboflavin (vitamin B_2), which inhibits the hepatocarcinogenesis caused solely by amino-azo dyes, and not by other carcinogens. This is due to the fact that the vitamin is a constituent of a flavin adenine dinucleotide, which behaves as an essential cofactor of the azo-reductase enzyme system (Kensler, 1949; Mueller and Miller, 1950; Rivlin, 1973). Clearly this is true only where N-hydroxylation of the intact amino-azo compound accounts for its hepatocarcinogenicity, and where the amine reduction products are not carcinogenic *per se*. It follows, in these cases, that animals on a high-flavin diet are at much lower risk of developing liver cancer from carcinogenic amino-azo dyes than animals with limited riboflavin.

Evidence at first sight suggests that selenium may function as another cofactor in the azo-reductase enzyme system, as the incorporation of 6 ppm of Se(Na_2SeO_3) in the drinking water of Sprague–Dawley rats exposed chronically to 3'-methyl-3-dimethylamino-azobenzene was found (Clayton and Baumann, 1949; Griffin and Jacobs, 1977) to reduce the incidence of liver tumours in 92% of the positive control rats to 46% of the pre-treated animals. Microsomal reductase activities are known to be increased by antioxidants, and the inhibition of tumour induction by selenium is more likely to be due to enhanced azo-reductase activity *per se* than to the presence of a possible cofactor. In many ways, selenium behaves as an antioxidant, like BHA, BHT and ethoxyquin (6-ethoxy-1,2-dihydro-2,2,4-trimethylquinoline) (3), which are also known to reduce the microsomal

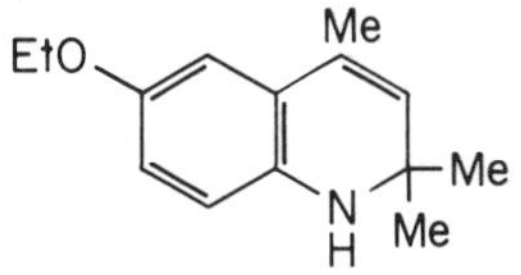

(3)

cytochrome P450 content (Batzinger, Ou and Bueding, 1978). This property helps to explain:

(*a*) The reduction of DEN-induced hepatocarcinogenesis in 100% of the positive control rats to only 27% of the animals, pre-treated with selenium (Dzhioev, 1978).
(*b*) The reduction of DEN-induced neoplasms in the lungs in 76% of the positive control mice to 54% of the animals, pre-treated with selenium (Dzhioev, 1978).
(*c*) The inhibitory effect of selenium on 1,2-dimethylhydrazine-induced tumours of the colon in rats (Jacobs, Jansson and Griffin, 1977; Dzhioev, 1978).

At present, the most plausible mechanism for the protective effects of the inducers of mixed function oxidases, antioxidants and inhibitors of cytochrome P450, invoke a disturbance in the balance between the metabolic activation of carcinogens and the detoxifying disposition of reactive carcinogen intermediates, and these mechanisms (q.v.) were stressed in the examples which have been cited in this section of the chapter. Mention has been made in addition of complications arising in the case of:

(*a*) Carcinogens which are direct acting and independent of metabolic activation.
(*b*) Carcinogens affecting extrahepatic sites.
(*c*) The involvement of inducers and inhibitors with carcinogens, which potentially affect several tissues, and can effect a shift of principal target organ.

The exposure of different susceptible tissues to chemical carcinogens by employing different administrative routes and different dosing regimens is well-known and, therefore, the importance of the biological events immediately following (carcinogen) dosing has been emphasized in those cases where the interpretation of the inhibition of tumour induction appears to be obscure.

Inhibition of tumour initiation by the interaction of nucleophiles with reactive carcinogen intermediates

In general, where inhibitory effects of tumour induction appear to be explicable in terms of a disturbance in the differential between metabolic activation of chemical carcinogens and the detoxifying disposition of reactive carcinogen intermediates, some contribution from direct interaction between inhibitor and the electrophilic species of ultimate carcinogens might be expected and at any rate cannot be altogether ruled out. Such a hypothetical interaction, which may operate in various circumstances to a very limited extent, would be hard to establish, but it seems to be particularly favoured where the inhibitor is either an RSH compound (*see below*) or where it provides a source of RSH compound(s) *in vivo* and, for example, disulphiram (1) is metabolized into N,N-diethyldithiocarbamate (2) and its S-glucuronide in mammals. It is feasible also that peroxide-scavenging hindered phenolic antioxidants, such as BHT (*Scheme 5.1*), may behave as nucleophiles with regard to alkylating molecular species (*Scheme 5.2*).

Entirely differently oriented studies (Jollow *et al.*, 1973, 1974a,b; Mitchell *et al.*, 1973a,b; Potter *et al.*, 1973, 1974; Zampaglione *et al.*, 1973; Mitchell and Jollow, 1975) have emphasized the protective role of the natural physiological metabolites, the cysteinyl peptides, and especially glutathione, that is played with regard to electrophilic species resulting from foreign compounds *in vivo*. In such a biological

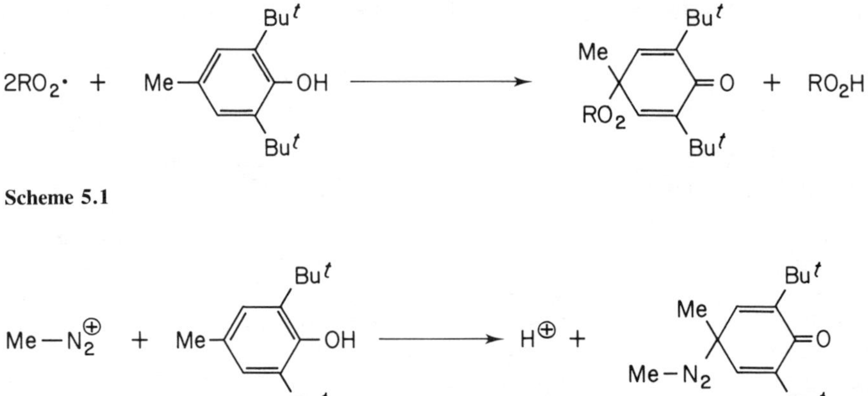

Scheme 5.1

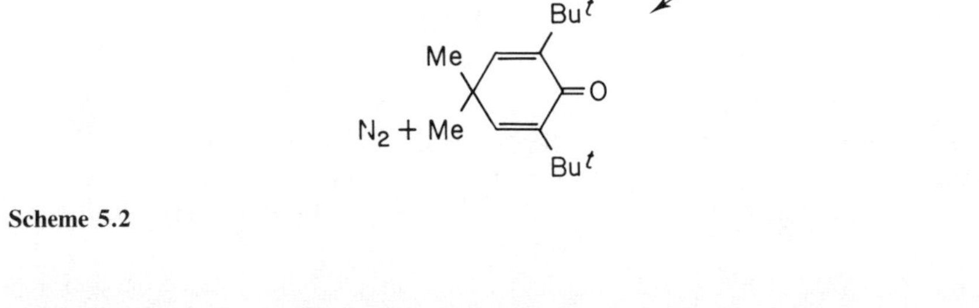

Scheme 5.2

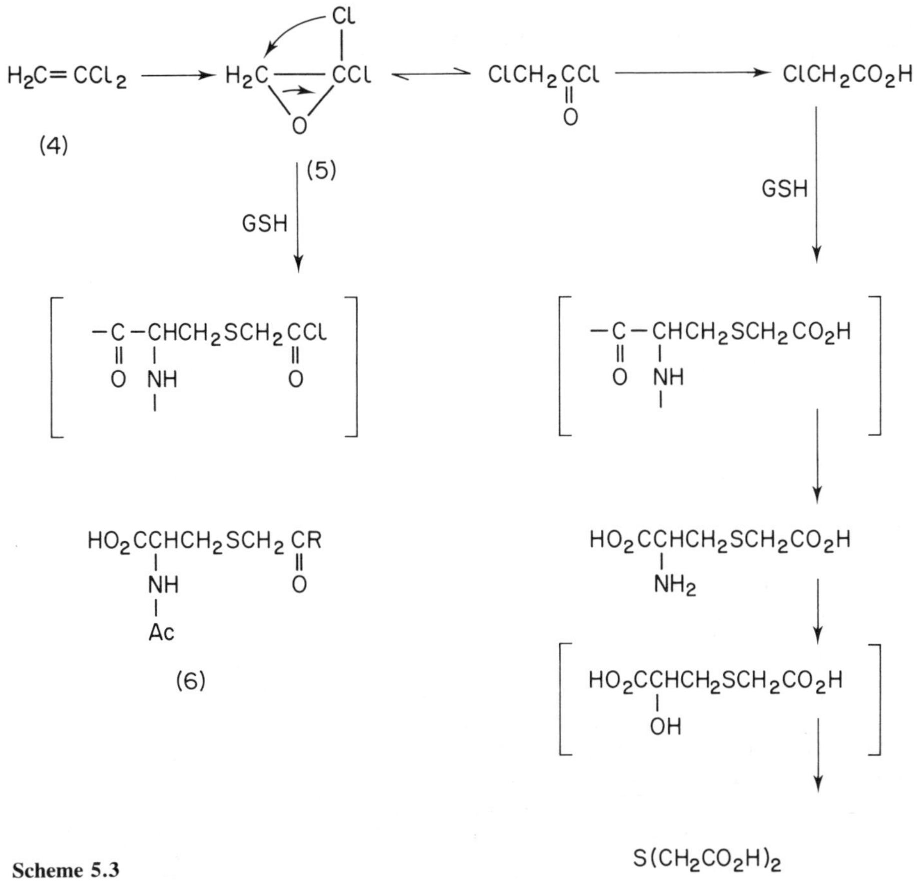

Scheme 5.3

$$H_2C=CCl_2 \longrightarrow H_2C\underset{O}{\overset{Cl}{-}}CCl \rightleftharpoons ClCH_2\underset{O}{\overset{\|}{C}}Cl \longrightarrow ClCH_2CO_2H$$

(4)   (5)

$$\left[\begin{array}{c} -C-CHCH_2SCH_2CCl \\ \| \ \ | \ \ \ \ \ \ \ \ \ \ \ \ \ \ \ \ \| \\ O \ \ NH \ \ \ \ \ \ \ \ \ \ \ \ O \\ | \end{array} \right] \quad \left[\begin{array}{c} -C-CHCH_2SCH_2CO_2H \\ \| \ \ | \\ O \ \ NH \\ | \end{array} \right]$$

$$\begin{array}{c} HO_2CCHCH_2SCH_2CR \\ | \| \\ NH \ \ \ \ \ \ \ \ \ \ \ \ \ \ \ O \\ | \\ Ac \end{array} \quad \begin{array}{c} HO_2CCHCH_2SCH_2CO_2H \\ | \\ NH_2 \end{array}$$

(6)

$$\left[\begin{array}{c} HO_2CCHCH_2SCH_2CO_2H \\ | \\ OH \end{array} \right]$$

$$S(CH_2CO_2H)_2$$

situation, the ultimate carcinogen metabolites would deplete cellular concentrations of cysteine, and so decrease glutathione biosynthesis. The mobilization of the hepatic pool of cysteine/glutathione to the assault of large doses of vinylidene chloride (4) provides a notable example of this, as its detoxifying metabolism along the two pathways (Scheme 5.3) is dependent on the glutathione available (Jones and Hathway, 1978a,b). In rats, 72% of a dose was metabolized, the remainder being excreted unchanged via the lungs, whereas, in mice, the higher activity of cytochrome P450 metabolizes 94% of the dose, and the difference in metabolism (22%) between the two species of animal is exactly matched by increased formation of the N-acetyl-S-cysteinylacetyl derivative (6) (28% in rats, 50% in mice). The proportion of the dose metabolized along the chloroacetic acid pathway is constant in the two species of animal. Whilst this demonstrates the capacity of the cysteine–glutathione pool to recognize and to accommodate different amounts of halogeno-olefine, glutathione, glutathione S-epoxide transferase and glutathione S-acid transferase do not compete entirely successfully with murine kidney- and liver-cell DNA for all of the 1,1-dichloroethylene oxide (5) produced. In mice, covalent binding to a kidney (and marginally to liver) DNA takes place, and compound (4) is carcinogenic to this species. Whether the concentration of cysteine–glutathione in murine kidney cells becomes rate limiting has not yet been

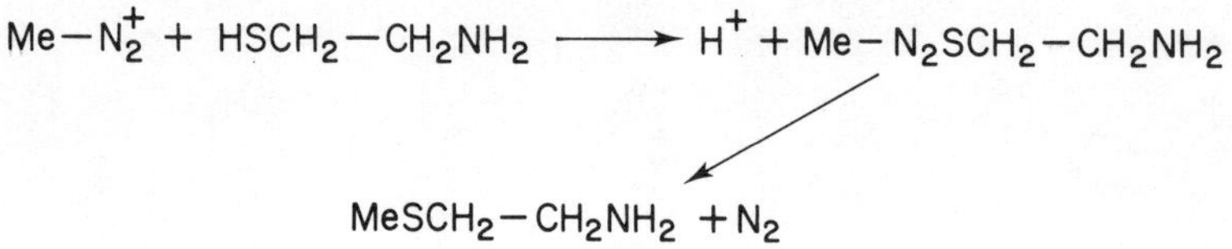

$$Me-N_2^+ + HSCH_2-CH_2NH_2 \longrightarrow H^+ + Me-N_2SCH_2-CH_2NH_2$$

$$MeSCH_2-CH_2NH_2 + N_2$$

Scheme 5.4

established. Nevertheless, vinylidene chloride is not mutagenic/carcinogenic in rats and in man (Jones and Hathway, 1978c), and in this regard cysteine–glutathione show(s) a remarkable inhibitory effect.

The protective effects of exogenous cysteamine against radiation injury are well-known. In the case of rats treated simultaneously with cysteamine and DMN, cysteamine appears to:

(a) React preferentially with the Me-N$_2^+$ alklylating species (*Scheme 5.4*).
(b) Reduce the formation of methyl analogues of the purine bases, including O^6-methylguanidine, in the liver DNA by more than 90% of that in positive control animals.
(c) Abolish the depression in liver-protein biosynthesis, which is produced by DMN alone (Kleihues, Margison and Margison, 1975; Pegg, 1977a).

The most likely inhibitors of tumour induction are undoubtedly the established metabolic inhibitors (like disulphiram) or inducers (like BHA, BHT etc.) of the detoxifying disposition of reactive intermediates, which can account for a whole dose of carcinogen and so act preventively, but substances like cysteamine, cysteine and glutathione, which react with carcinogenic electrophiles (*Schemes 5.3* and *5.4*), contribute substantial inhibitory effects. Incidentally, endogenous cysteamine is a starting material for taurine biosynthesis in mammals (Hirom and Millburn, 1981).

Hydroxyurea (7) is interesting in this context, as it protected KB cells specifically from assault by the direct-acting carcinogen MNNG (Aujard and Trincal, 1980).

$$HO-N-CNH_2 \longleftrightarrow HO-N=CNH_2$$

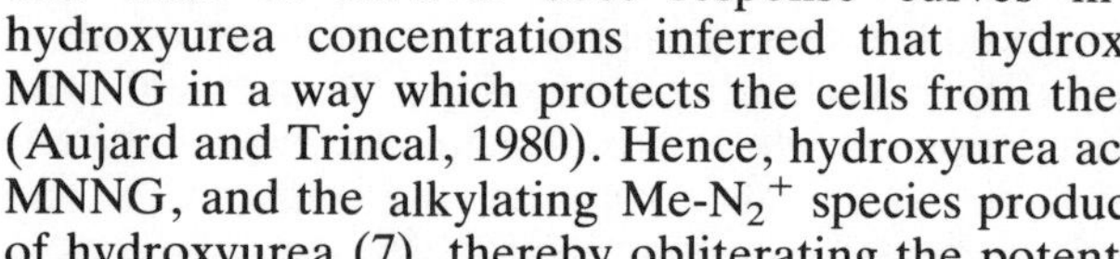

(7)

The shift of MNNG dose–response curves in the presence of increasing hydroxyurea concentrations inferred that hydroxyurea interacts directly with MNNG in a way which protects the cells from the toxic effect of the carcinogen (Aujard and Trincal, 1980). Hence, hydroxyurea accelerates the decomposition of MNNG, and the alkylating Me-N$_2^+$ species produced reacts with the enolic form of hydroxyurea (7), thereby obliterating the potentially toxic effect of unchanged MNNG (*Scheme 5.5*).

In other work, Yamshanov and Dzhioev (1981) have investigated the protective effect of exogenous nucleosides against alkylating carcinogens *in vivo*. Where either guanosine 200 µg g^{-1} or adenosine 180 µg g^{-1} was administered to rats 15 min before dosing labelled DMN, the extent of the Me-N$_2^+$ alkylation of the liver DNA was diminished significantly, and a similar result was obtained from experiments *in*

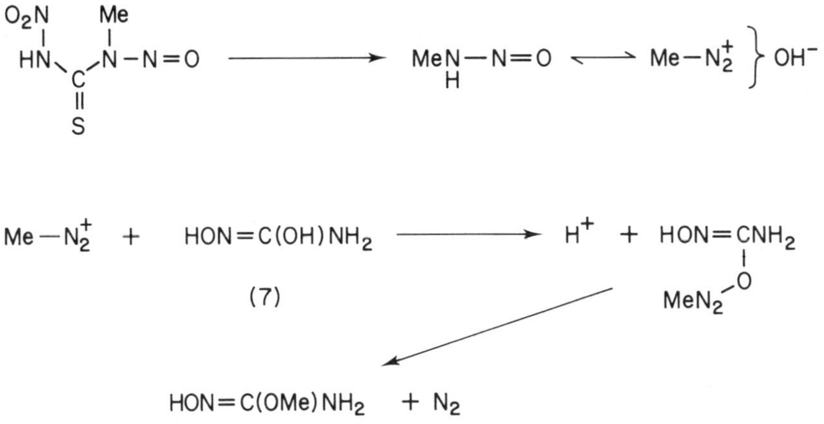

$$\underset{\substack{\text{HN}\diagdown\underset{\substack{\|\\S}}{C}\diagup}}{\overset{O_2N\quad Me}{\underset{|\quad\quad|}{\,}}}N-N=O \longrightarrow \underset{H}{MeN}-N=O \rightleftarrows \left.Me-N_2^+\right\}OH^-$$

$$Me-N_2^+ \;+\; HON=C(OH)NH_2 \longrightarrow H^+ \;+\; \underset{\underset{MeN_2}{|}}{HON=CNH_2}{\diagdown O}$$

(7)

$$HON=C(OMe)NH_2 \;+\; N_2$$

Scheme 5.5

vitro. Clearly, nucleophilic sites in the purine bases of the extracellular and extranuclear ribonucleosides competed successfully with those of the deoxyribonucleoside constituents of native DNA for the Me-N_2^+ alkylating species in the hepatocytes of living animals.

More complete evidence about the effect of exogenous nucleosides on animals exposed to DMN would be obtained through monitoring the (metabolic) fate of the administered nucleoside *per se* in addition to determining (Yamshanov and Dzhioev, 1981) their effect on the (level of) methylation of liver DNA. The new exercise might occasion the administration to rats of labelled nucleosides and unlabelled carcinogen, which Yamshanov and Dzhioev (1981) may have considered. Similarly, proper identification of the *S*-methylcysteamine reaction product would be valuable to Kleihues, Margison and Margison's work (1975).

It will be clear that some caution ought to be observed in attributing inhibitory effects to tumour induction to a direct interaction between the agent concerned and the electrophilic species resulting from ultimate carcinogens. The effect of administering large doses of ethionine (Pegg, 1977a) illustrates this point. Whilst this substance undoubtedly brings about (*a*) changes in the methylation pattern in rat-liver histones (Cox and Tuck, 1981), (*b*) increased transcriptional complexity and diminished enzymic methylation of DNA (Boehm and Drahowsky, 1981), and (*c*) alterations in replicational fidelity (Knaap, Glickman and Simons, 1981), competition occurs between *S*-adenosylethionine and *S*-adenosylmethionine and their interactions with the related methyltransferases and, in turn, with the cellular macromolecules DNA, RNA, histones etc. Accordingly, this is far from being a clearcut simple interaction, but it rather represents the competition of an analogue of a natural physiological metabolite with its natural counterpart in successive biological situations and systems.

Inhibition of tumour initiation through the induction of DNA-repair mechanisms

On the basis of all of the foregoing evidence (Chapters 2–5 inclusive), there is a strong supposition that the substitution of carcinogen-derived adducts at specific sites in the purine and pyrimidine residues belonging to the nucleotide pattern in DNA may lead to such semipermanent alterations in gene expression as are necessary for the initiation of multistage chemical carcinogenesis (Chapter 6). An important contribution to this proposition is made by those enzyme systems which implement the biological recognition and elimination of such promutagenic DNA lesions as substitutions and modification at O^6-position of guanine, and which may be present at various levels of activity in the several species, tissues and cell types that may be concerned.

In animals treated, for example, with alkylating carcinogens, certain organs, like the liver, appear to be much more resistant to tumorigenesis than the brain (Goth and Rajewsky, 1974) or the kidneys (Nicoll, Swann and Pegg, 1977). The conclusion is drawn that chemical carcinogenesis occurs where the level of activity of the recognitive and eliminative enzymes is low, i.e. where there are defective repair mechanisms. A good correlation between the persistence of specifically sited adducts in target-organ DNA (*see above*) and the occurrence of tumours (Pegg, 1977a) strongly supports this proposition.

The enzymic mechanisms which are responsible for the recognition and elimination of promutagenic lesions from DNA and the genetic control of these processes in mammalian cells have not yet been defined acceptably, but DNA glycosylases, endonucleases as well as des- and trans-alkylases are likely to be implicated (Laval, 1978; Lindahl, 1979). It is also feasible, however, that more than one such enzyme or that an enzyme with a totally different specificity is involved (Karran, Lindahl and Griffin, 1979). Some findings seem to infer that the enzymic activity responsible for removal of, say O^6-alkylguanine, from DNA may be inhibited by high concentrations of the carcinogens concerned, and possibly that it may be induced by chronic pre-treatment with small amounts of the same or of another agent (Nicoll, Swan and Pegg, 1975; Kleihues and Margison, 1976; Pegg, 1977b, 1978; Samson and Cairns, 1977; Montesano, Brésil and Margison, 1979; Robins and Cairns, 1979; Stumpf et al., 1979).

An agent which, administered to animals exposed to a carcinogen, brings about the excision of promutagenic lesions from target-organ DNA and DNA repair, would be of special interest in this context. It is envisaged that, primarily, such a substance would be an inducer of an endonuclease which is already present in the organ concerned, but at a low level of enzyme activity. It follows that the effects of partial hepatectomy would be relevant also in this connection, as the ensuing hyperplasia to redress the homeostasis of the organ is likely to induce the activities of various enzyme systems.

In the event, the activity of a hepatic endonuclease, which acts on double-stranded u.v.-irradiated and 2AAF-bound DNA, but not on double-stranded undamaged DNA, triples within 2 h of partial hepatectomy of rats (Van Lancker and Tomura, 1981). Interestingly, the endonuclease activity drops between 4 and 6 h after surgery, but remains at higher levels than those in non-hepatectomized rats until about 36 h after operation. Between 36 h and 2 days after surgery, the endonuclease activity in the partially hepatectomized rats falls below that of the non-hepatectomized ones, and then rises slowly to reach the levels found in non-hepatectomized rats between days 2 and 7 after operation (Van Lancker and Tomura, 1981). Studies of the effect of actinomycin D on the activity of crude enzymes and of the incorporation of [^{14}C]leucine and [^{14}C]valine into the purified enzyme indicate that the increase in enzymatic activity (*see above*) definitely results from *de novo* synthesis of endonuclease. Eighty per cent of endonucleolytic activity detectable in crude liver homogenates is inhibited by hyperimmune serum raised against the purified enzyme. Van Lancker and Tomura (1981) found that by adjusting the time of injection of [2-^{14}C]2AAF with respect to the levels of endonuclease activity after partial hepatectomy, an inverse relationship was established between DNA binding and enzyme activity.

On the other hand, in work involving a second chemical substance, Charlesworth et al. (1981) measured the levels of methylated purines in the kidney and liver DNA of rats, which had been pre-treated long-term with 2AAF in the diet, and which were then given single acute injections of DMN. In comparison with relevant control animals, the capacity of the livers of the pre-treated animals to remove O^6-methylguanine from hepatocyte DNA was greatly enhanced, but this did not apply to the renal DNA. Pre-treatment with 2AAF did not significantly affect the removal of either 3-methyladenine or 7-methyladenine from the liver DNA. The authors (Charlesworth et al., 1981) have clearly demonstrated, therefore, that an inducing agent like 2AAF may increase an animal's capacity to repair somatic DNA which is damaged in turn by a second chemical carcinogen. The mechanisms involved are uncertain, but it looks as though a hepatic endonuclease is implicated.

Two more points might be made. Firstly, clean repair of the damage caused to target-organ DNA by a carcinogen is as important as significant interference with its metabolism *in vivo* to the inhibition of tumour induction. The second point concerns the wide implications which the principles, established by Charlesworth et al. (1981), hold for mammals exposed to several different chemical substances.

Bibliography and references

AUJARD, C. and TRINCAL, G. (1980) *Carcinogenesis*, **1**(10), 819
BATZINGER, R.P., OU, S.-Y.L. and BUEDING, E. (1978) *Cancer Res.*, **38**, 4478
BECCI, P.J., THOMPSON, H.J., GRUBBS, C.J., SQUIRE, R.A., BROWN, C.C., SPORN, M.B. et al. (1978) *Cancer Res.*, **38**, 4463
BERENBLUM, I. (1929) *J. Pathol. Bacteriol.*, **32**, 425
BERENBLUM, I. (1941) *Cancer Res.*, **1**, 44
BERENBLUM, I. (1974) *Carcinogenesis as a Biological Problem*. pp. 41–49, 119–129 and 199–201. Amsterdam: North-Holland Publishing
BERRY, D.L., BRACKEN, W.R., SLAGA, T.J., WILSON, N.M., BUTTY, S.G. and JUCHAU, M.R. (1977) *Chem.-Biol. Interact.*, **18**, 129
BOEHM, T.L.J. and DRAHOVSKY, D. (1981) *Cancer Res.*, **41**, 4101
BUSK, L. and AHLBORG, U.G. (1980) *Toxicol. Lett.*, **6**(4–5), 243
CHA, Y.-N. and BUEDING, E. (1979) *Biochem. Pharmacol.*, **28**, 1917
CHARLESWORTH, J.D., CHU, Y.-H., O'CONNOR, P.J. and CRAIG, A.W. (1981) *Carcinogenesis*, **2**(4), 329
CLAYTON, C.C. and BAUMANN, G.A. (1949) *Cancer Res.*, **9**, 575
COX, R. and TUCK, M.T. (1981) *Cancer Res.*, **41**, 1253
CZYGAN, P., GREIM, H., GARRO, A.J., SCHAFFNER, F. and POPPER, H. (1974) *Cancer Res.*, **34**, 119
DIETRICH, R.A. and ERWIN, V.G. (1971) *Mol. Pharmacol.*, **7**, 301
DRUCKREY, H., PREUSSMANN, R., IVANKOVIC, S., SCHMIDT, C.H., MENNEL, H.D. and STAHL, K.W. (1964) *Z. Krebsforschung*, **66**, 280
DZHIOEV, F.K. (1978) *Kantserog N-Nitrozoedin: Deistire, Obraz. Opred., Mater. Simp*, 3rd edn. pp. 51–53
FIALA, E.S., BOBOTAS, G., KULAKIS, C. and WEISBURGER, J.H. (1977) *Xenobiotica*, **7**, 5
GOODMAN, J.I., TROSKO, J.E. and YAGER, J.D. (1976) *Chem.-Biol. Interact.*, **12**, 171
GOTH, R. and RAJEWSKY, M.F. (1974) *Proc. Natl Acad. Sci. USA*, **71**, 639
GRANTHAM, P.H., WEISBURGER, J.H. and WEISBURGER, E.K. (1973) *Food Cosmet. Toxicol.*, **11**, 209
GRIFFIN, A.C. and JACOBS, M.M. (1977) *Cancer Lett.*, **3**, 177
GRUBBS, C.J., MOON, R.C., SQUIRE, R.A., FARROW, G.M., STINSON, S.F., GOODMAN, D.G. et al. (1977) *Science*, **198**, 743
HATHWAY, D.E. (1966) *Adv. Food Res.*, **15**, 1

HIROM, P.C. and MILLBURN, P. (1981) In *Foreign Compound Metabolism in Mammals*. Ed. D.E. Hathway. Vol. 6. pp. 111–132. London: The Royal Society of Chemistry
IRVING, C.C., TICE, A.J. and MURPHY, W.M. (1979) *Cancer Res.*, **39**, 3040
ITO, N., MUTAYOSHI, K., MATSUMURA, K., DENDA, A., KANI, T., ARAI, M. et al. (1974) *Gann*, **65**, 123
JACOBS, M.M., JANSSON, B. and GRIFFIN, A.C. (1977) *Cancer Lett.*, **2**, 133
JOLLOW, D.J., MITCHELL, J.R., POTTER, W.Z., DAVIS, D.C., GILLETTE, J.R. and BRODIE, B.B. (1973) *J. Pharmacol. Exp. Ther.*, **187**, 195
JOLLOW, D.J., MITCHELL, J.R., ZAMPAGLIONE, N. and GILLETTE, J.R. (1974a) *Pharmacology*, **11**, 151
JOLLOW, D.J., THORGEIRSSON, S.S., POTTER, W.Z., HASHIMOTO, M. and MITCHELL, J.R. (1974b) *Pharmacology*, **12**, 251
JONES, B.K. and HATHWAY, D.E. (1978a) *Chem.-Biol. Interact.*, **20**, 27
JONES, B.K. and HATHWAY, D.E. (1978b) *Br. J. Cancer*, **37**, 411
JONES, B.K. and HATHWAY, D.E. (1978c) *Cancer Lett.*, **5**, 1
KARAMYSHEVA, A.F., KOBLYAKOV, V.A. and TURUSOV, V.S. (1980) *Eksp. Onkol.*, **2**(4), 50
KARRAN, P., LINDAHL, T. and GRIFFIN, B. (1979) *Nature*, **280**, 76
KENSLER, C.J. (1949) *J. Biol. Chem.*, **179**, 1079
KLEIHUES, P. and MARGISON, G.P. (1976) *Nature*, **259**, 153
KLEIHUES, P., MARGISON, J.M. and MARGISON, G.P. (1975) *Cancer Res.*, **35**, 3667
KNAAP, A.G.A.C., GLICKMAN, B.W. and SIMONS, J.W.I.M. (1981) *Mutat. Res.*, **82**(2), 355
LAM, L.K.T. and WATTENBERG, L.W. (1977) *J. Natl Cancer Inst.*, **58**, 413
LANG, M., MARSELOS, M. and TÖRRÖNEN, R. (1976) *Chem.-Biol. Interact.*, **15**, 267
LAVAL, J. (1978) *Biochimie*, **60**, 1123
LAWLEY, P.D. and THATCHER, C.J. (1970) *Biochem. J.*, **116**, 693
LINDAHL, T. (1979) *Prog. Nucleic Acid Res. Mol. Biol.*, **22**, 135
MALAMENT, D.S. and SHKLAR, G. (1981) *Carcinogenesis*, 2(8), 723
MARSELOS, M., LANG, M. and TÖRRÖNEN, R. (1976) *Chem.-Biol. Interact.*, **15**, 277
MATSUSHIMA, T., GRANTHAM, P.H., WEISBURGER, E.K. and WEISBURGER, J.H. (1972) *Biochem. Pharmacol.*, **21**, 2043
MEERMAN, J.H.N. and MULDER, G.J. (1981) *Life Sci.*, **28**, 2361
MEYSKENS, F.L. and PRASAD, K.N. (1983) *Modulation and Mediation of Cancer by Vitamins*. Basel: S. Karger
MITCHELL, J.R. and JOLLOW, D.J. (1975) In *Drugs and the Liver*. Eds. W. Gerok and K. Sicklinger. pp. 395–416. Stuttgart: Schattauer
MITCHELL, J.R., JOLLOW, D.J., POTTER, W.Z., DAVIS, D.C., GILLETTE, J.R. and BRODIE, B.B. (1973a) *J. Pharmacol. Exp. Ther.*, **187**, 185
MITCHELL, J.R., JOLLOW, D.J., POTTER, W.Z., GILLETTE, J.R. and BRODIE, B.B. (1973b) *J. Pharmacol. Exp. Ther.*, **187**, 211
MONTESANO, R., BRÉSIL, H. and MARGISON, G.P. (1979) *Cancer Res.*, **39**, 1798
MUELLER, G.C. and MILLER, J.A. (1950) *J. Biol. Chem.*, **185**, 145
NARISAWA, T., REDDY, B.S., WONG, C.W. and WEISBURGER, J.H. (1976) *Cancer Res.*, **36**, 1379
NICOLL, J.W., SWANN, P.F. and PEGG, A.E. (1975) *Nature*, **254**, 261
NICOLL, J.W., SWANN, P.F. and PEGG, A.E. (1977) *Chem.-Biol. Interact.*, **16**, 301
OKADO, M. (1976) In *Fundamentals in Cancer Prevention*. Eds P.N. Magee, S. Takayama and T. Sugimura. pp. 251–266. Baltimore: Baltimore University Park Press
OKADO, M. and ISHIDATE, M. (1977) *Xenobiotica*, **7**, 11
PEGG, A.E. (1977a) *Adv. Cancer Res.*, **25**, 195
PEGG, A.E. (1977b) *J. Natl Cancer Inst.*, **58**, 681
PEGG, A.E. (1978) *Nature*, **274**, 183
PERAINO, C., FRY, R.J.M. and STAFFELDT, E. (1971) *Cancer Res.*, **31**, 1506
PERAINO, C., FRY, R.J.M., STAFFELDT, E. and KISIELESKI, W. (1973) *Cancer Res.*, **33**, 2701
PERAINO, C., STAFFELDT, E.F., HAUGEN, D.A., LOMBARD, L.S., STEVENS, F.J. and FRY, R.J.M. (1980) *Cancer Res.*, **40**, 3268
POPPER, H., CZYGAN, P., GREIM, H., SCHAFFNER, F. and GARRO, A.J. (1973) *Proc. Soc. Exp. Biol. Med.*, **142**, 727
POTTER, W.Z., DAVIS, D.C., MITCHELL, J.R., JOLLOW, D.J., GILLETTE, J.R. and BRODIE, B.B. (1973) *J. Pharmacol. Exp. Ther.*, **187**, 203
POTTER, W.Z., THORGEIRSSON, S.S., JOLLOW, D.J. and MITCHELL, J.R. (1974) *Pharmacology*, **12**, 129
RIVLIN, R.S. (1973) *Cancer Res.*, **33**, 1977
ROBINS, P. and CAIRNS, J. (1979) *Nature*, **280**, 74
SAMSON, L. and CAIRNS, J. (1977) *Nature*, **267**, 281
SCHMÄHL, D., KRÜGER, F.W., HABS, M. and DIEHL, B. (1976) *Z. Krebsforschung*, **85**, 271

SCHULTZ, U. and McCALLA, D.R. (1969) *Can. J. Chem.*, **47**, 2021
SHAMBERGER, R.J., BAUGHMAN, F.F., KALCHERT, S.L., WILLIS, C.E. and HOFFMAN, G.C. (1973) *Proc. Natl Acad. Sci. USA*, **70**, 1461
SLAGA, T.J. and BRACKEN, W.R. (1977) *Cancer Res.*, **37**, 1631
SO, B.T., MAGADIA, N.E. and WYNDER, E.L. (1973) *J. Natl Cancer Inst.*, **50**, 927
STUMPF, R., MARGISON, G.P., MONTESANO, R. and PEGG, A.E. (1979) *Cancer Res.*, **39**, 50
TALALAY, P., BATZINGER, R.P., BENSON, A.M., BUEDING, E. and CHA, Y.-N. (1979) *Adv. Enzyme Regul.*, **17**, 23
ULLAND, B.M., WEISBURGER, J.H., YAMAMOTO, R.S. and WEISBURGER, E.K. (1972) *Toxicol. Appl. Pharmacol.*, **22**, 281
VAN LANCKER, J.L. and TOMURA, T. (1981) *Cancer Res.*, **41**, 2109
WATTENBERG, L. (1973) *J. Natl Cancer Inst.*, **50**, 1541
WATTENBERG, L.W. (1974) *J. Natl Cancer Inst.*, **52**, 1583
WATTENBERG, L.W. (1975) *J. Natl Cancer Inst.*, **54**, 1005
WATTENBERG, L.W. (1977) *J. Natl Cancer Inst.*, **58**, 395
WATTENBERG, L.W. (1980) *Cancer Res.*, **40**, 232
WEISBURGER, J.H. and WEISBURGER, E.K. (1973) *Pharmacol. Rev.*, **25**, 1
WYATT, P.L. and CRAMER, J.W. (1970) *Proc. Am. Assoc. Cancer Res.*, **11**, 83
YAMSHANOV, V.A. and DZHIOEV, F.K. (1981) *Vop. Onkol.*, **27**(2), 64
ZAMPAGLIONE, N., JOLLOW, D.J., MITCHELL, J.R., STRIPP, B., HAMRICK, M. and GILLETTE, J.R. (1973) *J. Pharmacol. Exp. Ther.*, **187**, 218
ZEMAITIS, M.A. and GREENE, F.E. (1976) *Biochem. Pharmacol.*, **25**, 1355

Chapter 6
Mechanisms in perspective: tumour promotion

On the basis of the evidence that was considered in the preceding chapter, a potentiation of tumour induction would be expected to result from (*a*) the induction of activating enzyme processes which generate reactive carcinogen intermediates, and (*b*) the inhibition of their detoxifying disposition, and this appears to be the case. Thus, whilst phenobarbital pre-treatment diminished 2AAF carcinogenicity in rats (Chapter 5), its administration after the carcinogen increased the incidence of 2AAF liver cancer (*see below*) in this species of animal (Peraino, Fry and Staffeldt, 1971; Peraino *et al.*, 1980). Similarly, phenobarbital administration after 3'-methyl-4-dimethylamino-azobenzene dosing increased the incidence of hyperblastic nodules attaching to the hepatocytes (Kaneko *et al.*, 1980). Clearly, promoters of hepatocarcinogenicity, which are inducers of hepatic drug-metabolizing enzymes *per se*, do not behave as cocarcinogens, for the simultaneous administration of carcinogen plus promoter increases the rate of carcinogen detoxication (Chapter 5) and decreases the incidence of tumours. On the other hand, the co-administration of benzo[a]pyrene and 1,1,1-trichloroprop-2-ene oxide to mice increased both the rate of appearance of skin tumours and their incidence (Karamysheva, Koblyakov and Turusov, 1980), by inhibiting epoxide hydratase and lowering the concentration of intracellular glutathione. 1,1,1-Trichloroprop-2-ene may properly be described as a cocarcinogen.

In addition to the foregoing means of potentiating tumour induction, the inhibition of DNA-repair processes would be expected to produce this result but, in practice, tumour promoters do not seem to cause unequivocal inhibition of DNA-repair synthesis. Thus, phorbol ester (TPA) neither inhibits repair in human amniotic cells after low doses of u.v. or 2AAF nor postreplicational repair in growing V79-4 Chinese hamster cells in response to u.v. irradiation (Trosko *et al.*, 1975). Such findings as these tend to separate the inhibition of DNA repair from mechanisms of tumour promotion, and the persistence of the initiating effect in the skin of the mice which had been treated with carcinogen prior to promotion with TPA, as well as the lack of correlation between the extent of tumour potentiation and the concentrations of promoter that are necessary to afford a standard degree of inhibition of repair (Gaudin, Gregg and Yielding, 1971, 1972), support this supposition. Other experiments, involving several cell types, show that tumour promoters inhibit normal DNA replication as much as or more than DNA-repair replication (Cleaver and Painter, 1975; Langenbach and Kuszynski, 1975; Poirier, De Cicco and Lieberman, 1975).

The preceding paragraphs attempt to account for the potentiation of tumour induction as far as this is possible in terms of the mechanisms that have been proposed. Difficulty arises, however, in interpreting experiments involving mouse skin, in which at least two distinct stages in chemical carcinogenesis, termed 'initiation' and 'promotion', have been recognized and the present narrative has hitherto been solely concerned with initiating chemical carcinogens that make stable modifications in the cellular genome (Chapter 3). In the mouse experiments, a single subthreshold dose of a DNA-damaging carcinogen may have been insufficient in itself to induce tumours, especially if a subsequent step or steps in a multistage process leading to cancer, were rate limiting. Unlike the carcinogens, promoters do not bind covalently to cellular DNA, and they are not mutagenic. Thus, since carcinogen was administered according to a two-stage regimen before the chronic application of promoter was begun, it is extremely unlikely that the combination of carcinogen plus promoter in the mouse experiments would have caused more extensive binding of the carcinogen to cellular DNA than would have occurred in the absence of promoter. Furthermore, there is no relationship between promotion and DNA repair (Cleaver and Painter, 1975; Langenbach and Kuszynski, 1975; Poirier, De Gicco and Lieberman, 1975). Hence, there is a strong suspicion that the actual action of promoters is entirely independent of that of initiating carcinogens, but that promoters act, at least in part, on the initiated cells.

Two-stage carcinogenesis in the skin system

A two-stage regimen for experiments concerned with promotion (*see above*) was first introduced by Mottram (1944), who produced skin tumours by treating the backs of mice with an acute subcarcinogenic dose of benzo[a]pyrene as initiator, followed by chronic application of croton oil (Berenblum, 1941). Initiation, which requires only a single administration of carcinogen, is thus a relatively rapid stage (Colburn and Boutwell, 1966), and it produces no apparent pathological change in the epidermis (Berenblum and Shubik, 1949; Scribner and Süss, 1978). On the other hand, promotion requires repeated topical applications (of promoter) over a period of several weeks and is accordingly a relatively slow stage (Berenblum and Shubik, 1947; Boutwell, 1964, 1974; Stenbäck, Garcia and Shubik, 1974). Clearly, the fact that promotion resulted in the induction of tumours shows that the preceding initiation had a lasting effect on the epidermis (Berenblum and Shubik, 1949; Scribner and Süss, 1978). That the epidermal cells appear to register the initiating event throughout an animal's life-span was established by Van Duuren *et al.* (1975) and Van Duuren, Smith and Melchionne (1978), who showed that exposure to a polycyclic aromatic hydrocarbon might be followed, after an interval of up to 56 weeks, by promotion with repeated topical applications of phorbol esters, and still result in the induction of skin tumours, despite the continuous renewal of the epidermis.

It would appear that the initiating carcinogen must be administered before the promoter in two-stage carcinogenicity experiments, and that tumour induction does not usually occur, if the order be reversed (Berenblum and Haran, 1955).

Whilst the action of the carcinogen is irreversible (Chapters 3, 4), that of promoters seems to be reversible, at any rate in the early stages of promotion. Thus, Boutwell (1964) showed that by increasing the intervals between successive applications of promoter beyond a certain optimal time, whilst keeping the size of aliquot doses and the cumulative dose of promoter constant, tumour induction in mouse skin was greatly reduced or even abolished. This implied that prolonged periods between treatment allowed reversion to take place. The fact that the termination of promotion, after benign tumours have begun to form, results in their regression, suggested that promotion may be reversible over a longer time scale than had been considered (Stenbäck, Garcia and Shubik, 1974). On the other hand, promotion can progress to the stage where the induction of malignant, non-regressing tumours seems to be inescapable. If promotion is ended just before tumours become evident, a smaller proportion of them will develop than would have been the case had chronic promoting treatment been continued (Burns *et al.*, 1978). Benign papillomas seem to represent the first evidence of tumours and, after further promoting treatment, malignant tumours appear, but it is uncertain whether they have developed from these papillomas (Burns *et al.*, 1978). Fürstenberger *et al.* (1981) have claimed to have resolved promotion into at least two separate steps.

TABLE 6.1. Tumour promotion by phorbol esters in tissues apart from mouse skin

Tissue	Mammalian species	Initiating carcinogen	Reference
Leukaemia	Mouse	7,12-Dimethylbenz[a]anthracene	Berenblum and Lonai (1970)
Liver and lungs	Mouse	DMN	Armuth and Berenblum (1972)
Leukaemia and mammary glands	Rat	7,12-Dimethylbenz[a]anthracene given by stomach tube	Armuth and Berenblum (1974)
Liver	Mouse	2AAF given transplacentally	Armuth and Berenblum (1977)
Intestine	Mouse	7,12-Dimethylbenz[a]anthracene or urethane given transplacentally	Goerttler and Loehrke (1977)
Forestomach	Mouse	7,12-Dimethylbenz[a]anthracene given intragastrically	Goerttler *et al.* (1979)
Glandular stomach	Rat	MNNG	Matsukura *et al.* (1979); Sugimura, Kawachi and Nakayasu (1978)
Oesophagus	Man	?	Weber and Hecker (1978)

Finally, in addition to mouse skin, other mammalian tissues are susceptible to the promotion of tumours by phorbol esters (*Table 6.1*). Thus, the parent diterpene alcohol of the phorbol ester series, viz. phorbol, which is not a promoter of the skin system *per se*, acts as a promoter of leukaemia and of tumours of the liver, lungs and mammary glands in carcinogen-initiated rodents (Berenblum and Lonai, 1970; Armuth and Berenblum, 1972, 1974, 1977). After topical application to mice, TPA promotes tumours in other organs (*Table 6.1*) as well as in the skin (Goerttler and Löehrke, 1976a,b, 1977), and after intragastric administration, tumour induction occurs in the forestomach of these animals (Goerttler *et al.*, 1979). Croton oil given freely to initiated rats in their drinking water promotes gastric carcinoma in the fundus or glandular part of the stomach (Sugimura, Kawachi and Nakayasu, 1978; Maksukura *et al.*, 1979).

The croton oil promoters

Two decades ago, Hecker *et al.* (Hecker, 1962; Hecker, Kubinyi and Bresch, 1964) and Van Duuren *et al.* (Van Duuren, Orris and Arroya, 1963; Van Duuren and

Orris, 1965) independently reported the isolation and characterization of the various tumour-promoting compounds from croton oil. All of these substances are esters of a parent compound phorbol, which had been isolated and partially characterized several years earlier (Flaschenträger, 1930; Flaschenträger and Falkenhausen, 1934; Flaschenträger and Wigner, 1942), and which was inactive in mouse skin *per se* (Baird and Boutwell, 1971; Hecker, 1971; Baird *et al.*, 1972). Detailed structural features of the several active phorbol esters were established by X-ray analysis of the appropriate bromo derivatives (Hoppe *et al.*, 1967; Pettersen and Ferguson, 1967), and stereochemical studies of the inter-related compounds were made by Crombie, Games and Pointer (1968). The most widely used phorbol ester, viz. phorbol myristate acetate, 12,*O*-tetradecanoylphorbol-13-acetate (TPA) (1) has the structure represented. Two major groups of phorbol esters have been identified; one of them has a long-chain ester group attached to C-12 (the A group)

(2), and the other one has a long-chain ester group attached to C-13 (the B group) (3). All of them contain one acid of chain length C_8–C_{16} and one of C_2–C_6. TPA is the most active phorbol ester, which has been tested in two-stage carcinogenicity experiments on mouse skin (Hecker, 1968, 1971; Van Duuren and Sivak, 1968; Van Duuren, 1969). Methods are available (Hecker, 1971) for the synthesis of both the A and B groups of phorbol esters from phorbol, prepared by hydrolysis of croton oil, and a great deal of attention has been given to the synthesis of symmetrical and unsymmetrical di-esters and to the assay of their promotional characteristics in two-stage experiments.

Tumour promoters for other physiological systems

The use of promoters, like the phorbol esters, has been extended to include several other structurally different substances with promoting activity (*Table 6.2*), in much the same way that the use of phorbol esters in the skin systems was applied to other physiological systems.

Anutrient sweeteners, such as cyclamate and saccharin, promote the induction of bladder tumours in rats, initiated with MNU (Hicks, Wakefield and Chowaniec, 1973, 1975; Hicks and Chowaniec, 1977; Hicks, 1980), and a number of the bile acids promote the induction of colon tumours in rats, initiated with MNNG (Narisawa *et al.*, 1974; Reddy *et al.*, 1976, 1977). DDT (Peraino *et al.*, 1975) and the polychlorinated biphenyls (PCBs) (Kimura, Kanematsu and Baba, 1976;

TABLE 6.2. Tumour promotion in rat tissues by substances other than phorbol esters

Tissue	Initiation	Promotion	Reference
Bladder	MNU, instilled in bladder	Saccharin, in diet	Hicks, Wakefield and Chowaniec (1973, 1975); Hicks and Chowaniec (1977)
Bladder	MNU, instilled in bladder	Cyclamate, in diet	Hicks, Wakefield and Chowaniec (1975); Hicks and Chowaniec (1977)
Colon	MNNG, intrarectally	Taurodeoxycholic acid, intrarectally	Narisawa *et al.* (1974)
Colon	MNNG, intrarectally	Lithocholic acid, intrarectally	Narisawa *et al.* (1974)
Colon	MNNG, intrarectally	Na deoxycholate, intrarectally	Reddy *et al.* (1976)
Colon	MNNG, intrarectally	Na cholate, intrarectally	Reddy *et al.* (1977)
Colon	MNNG, intrarectally	Na chenodeoxycholate, intrarectally	Reddy *et al.* (1977)
Liver	2AAF, in diet	DDT, in diet	Peraino *et al.* (1975)
Liver	3'-Me-DAB, in diet	PCBs, in diet	Kimura, Kanematsu and Baba (1976)
Liver	DEN, i.v. injection	PCBs, in diet	Nishizumi (1976)
Liver	2AAF, DAB, 3'-Me-DAB, in diet	Phenobarbital, in diet	Peraino, Fry and Staffeldt (1971); Peraino *et al.* (1973); Peraino, Fry and Grube (1978); Kitagawa and Sugano (1978)

Nishizuma, 1976) function as promoters in the liver system. Whilst phenobarbital undoubtedly induces the drug-metabolizing enzymes (Schulte-Hermann, 1974), it seems rather unlikely that this effect would account for its promoting activity with regard to hepatocarcinogenesis, especially as tumour induction is in fact inhibited by the co-administration of phenobarbital and carcinogen (Peraino, Fry and Staffeldt, 1971). Moreover, the promoting action of phenobarbital, in respect of liver tumours, operates in spacing experiments where several weeks were allowed to elapse between the administration of carcinogen and chronic treatment with the promoter (Peraino *et al.*, 1973).

Promoters cannot be used indiscriminately in any experimental model, and some of them appear to be tissue specific. Thus, for example, phorbol (Hecker, 1971; Baird, Melera and Boutwell, 1972; Slaga *et al.*, 1976), deoxycholic acid (Glauert and Bennink, 1978) and phenobarbital (Grube, Peraino and Fry, 1975) are inactive in the skin system, and as far as the present writer is aware, this also applies to cyclamate and saccharin.

The discovery of other promoters prompts the mention of some of the other experimental models of two-stage carcinogenesis.

Other experimental models of two-stage carcinogenesis

Bladder system

Hicks, Wakefield and Chowaniec (1973) first demonstrated that experimental bladder cancer might be separated into two stages. A single instillation of MNU into the bladder caused very few tumours, unless the animals (female rats) were maintained subsequently on a sodium cyclamate- or saccharin-containing diet (Hicks, Wakefield and Chowaniec, 1975; Hicks and Chowaniec, 1977). Cohen et al. (1979) replaced saccharin as promoter by *dl*-tryptophan in rats, which had been previously given N-[4-(5-nitro-2-furyl)-2-thioazolyl]formamide as initiator. The bladder model system was not so rigorously controlled as the skin had been (*see above*), but qualitatively different stages, modulated by different substances, were evident.

Similar spacing experiments to the ones which had demonstrated the persistence of the initiating effect in the case of the skin system, have been made in the experimental bladder (Cohen *et al.*, 1979). Where carcinogen-containing diet was followed 6 weeks later by a 5% saccharin diet, a 72% incidence of tumours resulted, compared with 95% where promotion followed straight after initiation. Where the carcinogen-containing diet was followed 6 weeks later by a tryptophan-rich diet, a 50% tumour incidence was obtained, compared with a 53% tumour incidence where promotion followed immediately after initiation.

It will be recalled that, after a subthreshold dose of an initiating carcinogen, the promotion of skin carcinogenesis required long-term chronic application of promoter (Berenblum, 1974), and that premature ending of promoter treatment permitted the regression of the papillary hyperplasia which had been stimulated. These findings seem to have been replicated in the bladder system. Thus, Arai, Cohen and Friedell (1977) demonstrated that chronic administration of cyclophosphamide was not carcinogenic to the rat bladder, but that long-term treatment (40 weeks) with cyclophosphamide did however promote the initiating effect of a threshold dose of N-[4-(5-nitro-2-furyl)-2-thioazolyl]formamide. The prolonged treatment with this weak promoter caused tumour induction in the bladder of 35% of the treated rats. Failure to promote tumour growth by multiple monthly doses of cyclophosphamide in the bladder of rats which had received a subthreshold dose of MNU, provides possible evidence for reversible promotion in the bladder system (Hicks, Gough and Walters, 1978).

Liver system

Islands of biochemically altered cells can be detected in the liver parenchyma long before a hepatocellular carcinoma is formed (Friedrich-Freksa, Gössner and Börner, 1969; Barnasch, 1976). Some of these island cells show a deficiency in specific enzymes, such as glucose-6-phosphatase and cannicular ATPase, some of them are glycogen deficient, and some of them have an increased glycogen content (Pitot *et al.*, 1978).

Phenobarbital does not induce the formation of islands in the liver parenchyma *per se* but, where it is given to animals after treatment with 2AAF or with another liver carcinogen, it increases the number and size of these foci, and it inhibits phenotypic reversion. This and other evidence (Kitigawa and Sugano, 1978) indicate that phenobarbital can promote carcinogen-altered cell populations into autonomous tumours.

Farber *et al.* (Farber, 1976; Solt and Farber, 1976; Solt, Medline and Farber, 1977) have described a model liver system in which DEN-initiated hepatocytes are stimulated selectively by a toxic growth inhibitor, for example a low level of 2AAF in the diet, followed by partial hepatectomy. The assumption is made that normal liver cells metabolically activate 2AAF into a metabolite which inhibits their growth, whereas the initiated or 'altered' cells are resistant (as they may have diminished capacity for metabolic activation), and they proliferate rapidly to form islands and hyperplastic nodules. The resistant cells can be stimulated to undergo at least 15 cycles of cell proliferation without giving evidence of autonomous growth: a late sign in their evolution to the cancer stage (Farber, 1976; Solt and Farber, 1976; Solt, Medline and Farber, 1977).

Clearly, as the foci of altered cells can be induced relatively rapidly by several structurally different hepatocarcinogens, the liver system (Farber, 1976) is a good model for studying the initiation of carcinogenesis. It would be more valuable still were the majority of these foci sensitive to promotion. As it is, only a small fraction of them develop into tumours, even under the pressure of cytotoxic exposure and partial hepatectomy (Solt, Medline and Farber, 1977).

Some criticism of the foregoing ideas might be timely at this point, in which case, the remainder of this chapter will be devoted to the problem of tumour promotion in the skin.

It may be relevant that the parenchymal island cells do not, in themselves, show ultimate signs, such as substantially increased mitotic rates or higher affinities for basophilic dyes, of their being tumour cells. Rather, at a much later stage in chemical carcinogenesis, when new cell populations have arisen within these islands, do cells with those properties begin to emerge, and they may possibly develop into liver tumours (Barnasch, 1976).

Another point concerns underlying theories of promotion of carcinogenesis based on (*a*) toxicity as the driving force, particularly in hepatocarcinogenesis; (*b*) the resistance of newly arising cell populations; (*c*) the selective advantage of such cells for tumour development. Thus, a single administration of carcinogen, in many cases, effects hepatocarcinogenesis *per se* and even in a model liver system, where the supply of chemical carcinogen can be critically regulated, a low yield of tumours is still produced. In which case, it may be difficult to understand how a carcinogen, which is by then absent, can (as it were) selectively pressurize liver-cell populations (Süss, 1984). It is perhaps relevant to consider that the size of a single dose of carcinogen which is used to produce tumours, is frequently unrealistically large. The resulting concentrations of reactive carcinogen intermediates *in vivo* would be sufficient to impair vital syntheses, to overwhelm the defence mechanisms of the target tissues, and to damage them so as to predispose them as effectively or more effectively towards tumour induction than would have been the case had smaller doses of carcinogen been used, followed by promotion.

Mode of action of tumour promotion in the skin

Investigations of the effects of TPA in cell culture suggested that (Van Duuren, 1969) the cell surface may be the primary target of attack by this promoter and, in further work (Fisher et al., 1979), a generalized change in the lipid phase of cell membranes has been demonstrated. This suggested that direct physicobiochemical action of TPA caused increased membrane fluidity. It became apparent in work with murine erythroleukaemia cells that growth in suspension was replaced by cellular adhesion to the tissue-culture plates within 30–120 min of exposure to TPA (Yamasaki et al., 1979). The induction of this adhesivity or 'stickiness' (Lowe, Pacifici and Holtzer, 1978; Castagna, Rochette-Egly and Rosenfeld, 1979; Yamasaki et al., 1979) is considered to be very important to cellular mechanisms leading to tumour induction (see below). Another early cellular response to TPA treatment was the release of arachidonic acid from the membrane phospholipids (Mufson, De Feo and Weinstein, 1979), which was supposed to be associated with stimulation of prostaglandin biosynthesis.

In general, chemical compounds produce biological responses through existing physiological mechanisms, and it was considered that TPA may be concerned with processes of growth regulation or hormonal activity. A number of observations (Lee and Weinstein, 1978a) apparently supported this supposition. Thus, originally, epidermal polypeptide hormone (EGF) was considered to be an endogenous substance that may be involved and, in support of this supposition, both EGF and TPA had been shown to be plasminogen activators in HeLa-cell cultures (Castro, Pieczynski and Di Paolo, 1973). A considerable body of evidence (Lee and Weinstein, 1978b, 1979; Todaro and DeLarco, 1978; Brown, Dicker and Rozengurt, 1979) showed, however, that in effect TPA inhibited EGF binding by indirectly changing the conformation of EGF receptors. In this connection, such conformational changes occur also in the functioning of other hormone receptors (De Meyts, Bianco and Roth, 1976; Singer, 1976; Das and Fox, 1978; Schlessinger et al., 1978), and are reminiscent of the allosteric modification of the globin protein that accounts for the sigmoid O_2 saturation curve for haemoglobin (Hathway, 1984).

Thus, whilst promoters appeared to act primarily on receptors associated with cell membranes, which would seem to account in part for their unique physiological function, it was uncertain how this happened. Recent work (Weinstein, 1981; Castagna et al., 1982; Ashendel, Staller and Boutwell, 1983; Kraft and Anderson, 1983; Niedel, Kuhn and Vandenbark, 1983) has shown the mode of action of TPA to involve a specific calcium-dependent and lipid-dependent protein kinase enzyme system, viz. protein kinase C. Thus, for example, TPA plus phospholipid increases the activity of protein kinase C. Induced changes in lipid structure might, in the presence of Ca^{2+}, increase the binding of phospholipid to protein kinase C apoprotein, and this would seem to explain why protein kinase C appears to be transported from the cytosol to the membranes where cells were treated with TPA (Kraft and Anderson, 1983). Hydrophilic regions associated with TPA might also interact in some way with protein kinase C apoprotein to increase formation of phospholipid–protein kinase C–TPA–Ca^{2+} complex. Hence, the exposure of cells to TPA increased the turnover of membrane phospholipid, which generated, in turn, diacetylglycerol (Castagna et al., 1982), which would further amplify the activity of protein kinase C. Thus, in this sense, diacetylglycerol behaved as a putative endogenous analogue of the tumour promoters (Weinstein, 1981, 1983).

This is an important discovery, as the well-known effect of dietary fat in potentiating carcinogenesis may be attributed to a modification of membrane surface properties in such a way as to influence protein kinase activities.

A number of other effects of TPA, which require RNA and protein biosynthesis, seem to reflect the so-called 'transmembrane signals' on cytoplasmic and nuclear functions. In the case of TPA, these responses include the induction of plasminogen activator synthesis (Wigler and Weinstein, 1976; Weinstein, Wigler and Pietropaolo, 1977; Weinstein et al., 1978; Wigler, De Feo and Weinstein, 1978) and of ornithine decarboxylase synthesis (Bowden et al., 1975; O'Brien, Simsiman and Boutwell, 1975a,b, 1976; O'Brien and Diamond, 1977). There must also be included in this category of responses the inhibition or potentiation of DNA biosynthesis, as well as effects on the expression of terminal differentiation (Berenblum, 1954), and some observations on mouse skin support this supposition (Raick, 1974; Colburn, Law and Head, 1975; Yuspa et al., 1976). Furthermore, the evidence provided by work involving cell-culture systems (Cohen et al., 1977; Diamond, O'Brien and Rovera, 1977; Pacifici and Holtzer, 1977; Rovera, O'Brien and Diamond, 1977; Yamasaki et al., 1977; Ishii et al., 1978; Mufson, Fisher and Weinstein, 1978) showed that phorbol esters can powerfully influence terminal differentiation. There is a strong supposition (Weinstein et al., 1979) that this effect is also very important to the mode of action of tumour promotion.

From the pathological point of view, which is important to tumorigenesis, cells of the epidermis originate in the basal layer and ascend to the so-called differentiated layer of cells and ultimately into the stratum corneum or horny external layer of the epidermis from which dead cells are continuously discarded. Whilst the basal (stem) cells are continuously dividing, homeostasis is maintained with a stable pool of basal cells. Apparently, immediately after cell division, mother and daughter-cells remain in the basal layer and a neighbouring cell is pushed up indirectly into the differentiated layer of cells (Potten and Allen, 1975; Fürstenburger et al., 1981). If one of the cells in the basal layer be assumed to be a protumour or tumour cell, it would also participate in cell division and in the pushing process. Both the daughter-cells of normal and tumour cells would pass through the layers of differentiated cells into the horny external layer from which eventually they would be discarded. Evidence at first sight would suggest that, even if tumour cells divide at a slightly faster rate than the normal ones, they would be unlikely to form a tumour in this biological situation, where all of the daughter-cells are facilely discarded.

Another factor which may contribute to the situation where a population of latent tumour cells is increasing with time, is the increased 'stickiness' of latent tumour cells compared with normal cells (Süss, 1984). If latent tumour cells were more 'sticky' than normal ones, and in fact it looks as though this is the case (Yamasaki et al., 1979; Weinstein, 1981), they would be harder to push up into the other dividing cells and, in the long run, the population of cells in the basal layer would change from normal, less 'sticky' cells to protumour, 'stickier' ones. On the other hand, a further model (Weinstein et al., 1979) emphasized that basal cell division might be interrupted by the action of promoter, and the initiated protumour cell might undergo exponential cell division to afford a clone of similar cells. As TPA is supposed to be able to induce phenotypic changes in cells which mimic transported ones, the environment of a clone of such cells might increase their outgrowth per se, and influence their development into a tumour.

Whilst different cell populations are detectable in hepatocarcinogenesis (Farber,

1979), latent tumour cells, which are tacitly assumed to develop, have never been identified in the skin. It is well-known that normal cells are transformed into tumour cells by chemical carcinogens (Berward and Sachs, 1965), and the observed difference between the liver and skin systems makes the problem of tumour promotion in skin more intangible.

Nevertheless, the skin system facilitated the discovery of different stages in chemical carcinogenesis, and the assumption might be made that a full dose of carcinogen acts as initiator and promoter. Alternatively, where exogenous promoter is not employed, it is now tempting to speculate that the properties of proliferating carcinogen-initiated cells may be modified through the action of endogenous promoters, such as diacetylglycerol, on membrane-associated receptors.

It will be recalled that, in the early stages of promotion by TPA, regenerative processes can occur in the time intervals in spacing experiments, but this is untrue for carcinogens. In fact, if a carcinogen, such as 7,12-dimethylbenz[a]anthracene, be painted on the mouse skin with increasing periods of time between successive applications, the yield of tumours may even be increased (Cramer and Stowell, 1941; Süss, 1984). Thus, 'reversible promotion' seems to be independent of an initiating event, and may relate to similarly induced effects in populations of normal cells.

In conclusion, a simple picture of cellular recognition and initiation and of rapidly proliferating mutant cells within the economy of a target organ, leading to tumour induction under the influence of various promoters and physiological factors, seems to be consistent with the accumulated evidence. The mode of action of promoters appears to be specifically concerned with (a) the general modification of the cell surface properties through its interaction with a receptor associated with cell membranes, viz. with protein kinase C, which makes protumour cells become more 'sticky', as well as with (b) the rapid proliferation of these protumour cells. Other parameters, such as genetic redistribution which takes place (Chapter 7), may contribute also to tumour promotion/induction, but the general framework of biological events leading to tumour induction, which has been discussed, is unlikely to change very much with future progress. In particular, the recognitive and initiating biological events (Chapters 2–4) are held to be very important to the subsequent changes, irrespective of whether somatic DNA as a whole or specific oncogenes (Chapter 7) be implicated. The contemporary state of awareness and understanding concerning the mode of action of tumour promotion has helped to eliminate much of the mystery from the important processes which are concerned.

Bibliography and references

ARAI, M., COHEN, S.M. and FRIEDELL, G.H. (1977) *Proceedings of the 36th Annual Meeting of the Japanese Cancer Association*, Tokyo, Oct. 1977. Gann (Suppl.), p. 39
ARMUTH, V. and BERENBLUM, I. (1972) *Cancer Res.*, **32**, 2259
ARMUTH, V. and BERENBLUM, I. (1974) *Cancer Res.*, **34**, 2704
ARMUTH, V. and BERENBLUM, I. (1977) *Int. J. Cancer*, **20**, 292
ASHENDEL, C.L., STALLER, J.M. and BOUTWELL, R.K. (1983) *Biochem. Biophys. Res. Commun.*, **111**, 340
BAIRD, W.M. and BOUTWELL, R.K. (1971) *Cancer Res.*, **31**, 1074
BAIRD, W.M., MELERA, P.W. and BOUTWELL, R.K. (1972) *Cancer Res.*, **32**, 781
BARNASCH, P. (1976) *Cancer Res.*, **36**, 2555
BERENBLUM, I. (1941) *Cancer Res.*, **1**, 807
BERENBLUM, I. (1954) *Adv. Cancer Res.*, **2**, 129
BERENBLUM, I. (1974) *Carcinogenesis as a Biological Problem*. Amsterdam: North-Holland

BERENBLUM, I. and HARAN, N. (1955) *Br. J. Cancer*, **9**, 268
BERENBLUM, I. and LONAI, V. (1970) *Cancer Res.*, **30**, 2744
BERENBLUM, I. and SHUBIK, P. (1947) *Br. J. Cancer*, **1**, 379
BERENBLUM, I. and SHUBIK, P. (1949) *Br. J. Cancer*, **3**, 384
BERWARD, Y. and SACHS, L. (1965) *J. Natl Cancer Inst.*, **35**, 641
BOUTWELL, R.K. (1964) *Prog. Exp. Tumor Res.*, **4**, 207
BOUTWELL, R.K. (1974) *CRC Critical Rev. Toxicol.*, **2**, 419
BOWDEN, G.T., TROSKO, J.E., SHAPAS, B.G. and BOUTWELL, R.K. (1975) *Cancer Res.*, **35**, 3599
BROWN, K.D., DICKER, P. and ROZENGURT, E. (1979) *Biochem. Biophys. Res. Commun.*, **86**, 1037
BURNS, F.J., VANDERLAAN, M., SNYDER, E. and ALBERT, R.E. (1978) In *Carcinogenesis*. Vol. 2: *Mechanisms of Tumor Promotion and Cocarcinogenesis*. Eds T.J. Slaga, A. Sivak and R.K. Boutwell. pp. 91–96. New York: Raven Press
CASTAGNA, M., ROCHETTE-EGLY, C. and ROSENFELD, C. (1979) *Cancer Lett.*, **6**, 227
CASTAGNA, M., TAKAI, Y., KAIBUCHI, K., SANO, K., KIKAWA, U. and NISHIZUKA, Y. (1982) *J. Biol. Chem.*, **257**, 7847
CASTRO, B.C., PIECZYNSKI, W.J. and DI PAOLO, J.A. (1973) *Cancer Res.*, **33**, 819
CLEAVER, J.E. and PAINTER, R.B. (1975) *Cancer Res.*, **35**, 1773
COHEN, R., PACIFICI, M., RUBENSTEIN, N., BIEHL, J. and HOLTZER, H. (1977) *Nature*, **266**, 538
COHEN, S.M., ARAI, M., JACOBS, J.B. and FRIEDELL, G.H. (1979) *Cancer Res.*, **39**, 1207
COLBURN, N.H. and BOUTWELL, R.K. (1966) *Cancer Res.*, **26**, 1701
COLBURN, N.H., LAW, S. and HEAD, R. (1975) *Cancer Res.*, **35**, 3154
CRAMER, W. and STOWELL, R.E. (1941) *Cancer Res.*, **1**, 849
CROMBIE, L., GAMES, M. and POINTER, D.J. (1968) *J. Chem. Soc.*, **C**, 1347
DAS, M. and FOX, C.F. (1978) *Proc. Natl Acad. Sci. USA*, **75**, 2644
DE MEYTS, P., BIANCO, A.R. and ROTH, J. (1976) *J. Biol. Chem.*, **251**, 1877
DIAMOND, L., O'BRIEN, T.G. and ROVERA, G. (1977) *Nature*, **269**, 247
FARBER, E. (1976) In *Liver Cell Cancer*. Eds H.M. Cameron, D.A. Linsell and G.P. Warwick. pp. 243–277. Amsterdam: Elsevier
FARBER, E. (1979) *Adv. Cancer Res.*, **31**, 125
FISHER, P.B., FLAMM, M., SCHACHTER, D. and WEINSTEIN, I.B. (1979) *Biochem. Biophys. Res. Commun.*, **86**, 1063
FLASCHENTRÄGER, B. (1930) *Z. Angew. Chem.*, **43**, 1011
FLASCHENTRÄGER, B. and FALKENHAUSEN, F.V. (1934) *Justus Liebigs Annln. Chem.*, **514**, 252
FLASCHENTRÄGER, B. and WIGNER, G. (1942) *Helv. Chim. Acta.*, **25**, 569
FRIEDRICH-FREKSA, H., GÖSSNER, W. and BÖRNER, P. (1969) *Z. Krebsforschung*, **72**, 226
FÜRSTENBERGER, G., BERRY, D.L., SORG, B. and MARKS, F. (1981) *Proc. Natl Acad. Sci. USA*, **78**, 7722
GAUDIN, D., GREGG, R.S. and YIELDING, K.L. (1971) *Biochem. Biophys. Res. Commun.*, **45**, 630
GAUDIN, D., GREGG, R.S. and YIELDING, K.L. (1972) *Biochem. Biophys. Res. Commun.*, **48**, 945
GLAUERT, H.P. and BENNINK, M.R. (1978) *Res. Commun. Chem. Pathol. Pharmacol.*, **22**, 609
GOERTTLER, K. and LOEHRKE, H. (1976a) *Virchows Arch. pathol. Anat. Physiol.*, **370**, 97
GOERTTLER, K. and LOEHRKE, H. (1976b) *Virchows Arch. pathol. Anat. Physiol.*, **372**, 29
GOERTTLER, K. and LOEHRKE, H. (1977) *Virchows Arch. pathol. Anat. Physiol.*, **376**, 117
GOERTTLER, K., LOEHRKE, H., SCHWEIZER, J. and HESSE, B. (1979) *Cancer Res.*, **39**, 1293
GRUBE, D.D., PERAINO, C. and FRY, R.J.M. (1975) *J. Invest. Dermatol.*, **64**, 258
HATHWAY, D.E. (1984) *Molecular Aspects of Toxicology*. Chap. 9. London: The Royal Society of Chemistry
HECKER, E. (1962) *Angew. Chem.*, **74**, 722
HECKER, E. (1968) *Cancer Res.*, **28**, 2338
HECKER, E. (1971) In *Methods in Cancer Research*. Ed. H. Busch. Vol. 6, pp. 439–484. New York: Academic Press
HECKER, E., KUBINYI, H. and BRESCH, H. (1964) *Angew. Chem. Int. Edn*, **3**, 747
HICKS, R.M. (1980) *Br. Med. Bull.*, **36**, 39
HICKS, R.M. and CHOWANIEC, J. (1977) *Cancer Res.*, **37**, 2943
HICKS, R.M., GOUGH, T.A. and WALTERS, C.L. (1978) In *Environmental Aspects of N-Nitroso Compounds*. International Agency for Research on Cancer Scientific Publications, no. 19. Eds E.A. Walker, M. Castegnaro, L. Griciute and R.E. Lyle. pp. 465–475. Lyon, France: IARC
HICKS, R.M., WAKEFIELD, J.ST.J. and CHOWANIEC, J. (1973) *Nature*, **243**, 347
HICKS, R.M., WAKEFIELD, J.ST.J. and CHOWANIEC, J. (1975) *Chem.-Biol. Interact.*, **11**, 225
HOPPE, W., BRANDL, F., STRELL, I., RÖHRL, M., GASSMANN, J., HECKER, E. *et al.* (1967) *Angew. Chem.*, **79**, 824
ISHII, D.N., FIBACH, E., YAMASAKI, H. and WEINSTEIN, I.B. (1978) *Science*, **200**, 556

KANEKO, A., DEMPO, K., KAKU, T., YOKOYAMA, S., SATOH, M., MORI, M. et al. (1980) *Cancer Res.*, **40**, 1658
KARAMYSHEVA, A.F., KOBLYAKOV, V.A. and TURUSOV, V.S. (1980) *Eksp. Onkol.*, **2**(4), 50
KIMURA, N.T., KANEMATSU, T. and BABA, T. (1976) *Z. Krebsforschung*, **87**, 257
KITAGAWA, T. and SUGANO, H. (1978) *Gann*, **69**, 679
KRAFT, A.S. and ANDERSON, W.B. (1983) *Nature*, **301**, 621
LANGENBACH, R. and KUSZYNSKI, C. (1975) *J. Natl Cancer Inst.*, **55**, 801
LEE, L.S. and WEINSTEIN, I.B. (1978a) *Science*, **202**, 313
LEE, L.S. and WEINSTEIN, I.B. (1978b) *Nature*, **274**, 696
LEE, L.S. and WEINSTEIN, I.B. (1979) *J. Cell Physiol.*, **99**, 451
LOWE, M.E., PACIFICI, M. and HOLTZER, H. (1978) *Cancer Res.*, **38**, 2350
MATSUKURA, N., KAWACHI, T., SANO, T., SASAJIMA, K. and SUGIMURA, T. (1979) *J. Cancer Res. Clin. Oncol.*, **93**, 323
MOTTRAM, J.C. (1944) *J. Pathol. Bacteriol.*, **56**, 181
MUFSON, R.A., DE FEO, D. and WEINSTEIN, I.B. (1979) *Mol. Pharmacol.*, **16**, 569
MUFSON, R.A., FISHER, P.B. and WEINSTEIN, I.B. (1978) *Proc. Am. Assoc. Cancer Res.*, **19**, 183
NARISAWA, T., MAGADIA, N.E., WEISBURGER, J.H. and WYNDER, E.L. (1974) *J. Natl Cancer Inst.*, **53**, 1093
NIEDEL, J.E., KUHN, L.J. and VANDENBARK, G.R. (1983) *Proc. Natl Acad. Sci. USA*, **80**, 36
NISHIZUMI, M. (1976) *Cancer Lett.*, **2**, 11
O'BRIEN, T.G. and DIAMOND, L. (1977) *Cancer Res.*, **37**, 3895
O'BRIEN, T.G., SIMSIMAN, R.C. and BOUTWELL, R.K. (1975a) *Cancer Res.*, **35**, 1662
O'BRIEN, T.G., SIMSIMAN, R.C. and BOUTWELL, R.K. (1975b) *Cancer Res.*, **35**, 2426
O'BRIEN, T.G., SIMSIMAN, R.C. and BOUTWELL, R.K. (1976) *Cancer Res.*, **36**, 3766
PACIFICI, M. and HOLTZER, H. (1977) *Am. J. Anat.*, **150**, 207
PERAINO, C., FRY, R.J.M. and GRUBE, D.D. (1978) In *Carcinogenesis. Vol. 2: Mechanisms of Tumor Promotion and Cocarcinogenesis*. Eds T.J. Slaga, A. Sivak and R.K. Boutwell. pp. 421–432. New York: Raven Press
PERAINO, C., FRY, R.J.M. and STAFFELDT, E. (1971) *Cancer Res.*, **31**, 1506
PERAINO, C., FRY, R.J.M., STAFFELDT, E. and CHRISTOPHER, J.P. (1975) *Cancer Res.*, **35**, 2884
PERAINO, C., FRY, R.J.M., STAFFELDT, E. and KISIELESKI, W.E. (1973) *Cancer Res.*, **33**, 2701
PERAINO, C., STAFFELDT, E.F., HAUGEN, D.A., LOMBARD, L.S., STEVENS, F.J. and FRY, R.J.M. (1980) *Cancer Res.*, **40**, 3268
PETTERSEN, R.C. and FERGUSON, G. (1967) *Chem. Commun.*, 716
PITOT, H.C., BARSNESS, L., GOLDSWORTHY, T. and KITAGAWA, T. (1978) *Nature*, **271**, 456
POIRIER, M.C., DE CICCO, B.T. and LIEBERMAN, M.W. (1975) *Cancer Res.*, **35**, 1392
POTTEN, C.S. and ALLEN, T.D. (1975) *Differentiation*, **3**, 161
RAICK, A.N. (1974) *Cancer Res.*, **34**, 2915
REDDY, B.S., NARASAWA, T., WEISBURGER, J.H. and WYNDER, E. (1976) *J. Natl Cancer Inst.*, **56**, 441
REDDY, B.S., WATANABE, J., WEISBURGER, J.H. and WYNDER, E. (1977) *Cancer Res.*, **37**, 3238
ROVERA, G., O'BRIEN, T.G. and DIAMOND, L. (1977) *Proc. Natl Acad. Sci. USA*, **74**, 2894
SCHLESSINGER, J., SCHECHTER, Y., CUATRECASAS, P., WILLINGHAM, M.C. and PASTAN, I. (1978) *Proc. Natl Acad. Sci. USA*, **75**, 5353
SCHULTE-HERMANN, R. (1974) *CRC Crit. Rev. Toxicol.*, **3**, 97
SCRIBNER, J.D. and SÜSS, R. (1978) In *International Review of Experimental Pathology*. Eds G.W. Richter and M.A. Epstein. Vol. 43. pp. 137–198. New York: Academic Press
SINGER, S.J. (1976) In *Surface Membrane Receptors*. Eds R.A. Bradshaw, W.A. Frazier, R.C. Merrell, D.I. Gottlieb and R.A. Hogue-Angelitti. pp. 1–24. New York: Plenum Press
SLAGA, T.J., SCRIBNER, J.D., THOMPSON, S. and VIAJE, A. (1976) *J. Natl Cancer Inst.*, **57**, 1145
SOLT, D. and FARBER, E. (1976) *Nature*, **263**, 701
SOLT, D., MEDLINE, A. and FARBER, E. (1977) *Am. J. Pathol.*, **88**, 595
STENBÄCK, F., GARCIA, H. and SHUBIK, P. (1974) In *The Physiopathology of Cancer*, 2nd edn. pp. 517–562. New York: Hoebner-Harper
SUGIMURA, T., KAWACHI, T. and NAKAYUSA, N. (1978) In *Abstracts of Papers, Cold Spring Harbor Meeting*. p. 30. Cold Spring Harbor Laboratory, Cold Spring Harbor, New York
SÜSS, R. (1984) In *Molecular Aspects of Toxicology*. Ed. D.E. Hathway. Chap. 12. London: The Royal Society of Chemistry
TODARO, G. and DELARCO, J.G. (1978) *Cancer Res.*, **38**, 4147
TROSKO, J.E., YAGER, J.D., BOWDEN, G.T. and BUTCHER, F.R. (1975) *Chem.-Biol. Interact.*, **11**, 191
VAN DUUREN, B.L. (1969) *Prog. Exp. Tumor Res.*, **11**, 31
VAN DUUREN, B.L. and ORRIS, L. (1965) *Cancer Res.*, **25**, 1871
VAN DUUREN, B.L., ORRIS, L. and ARROYA, E. (1963) *Nature*, **200**, 1115
VAN DUUREN, B.L. and SIVAK, A. (1968) *Cancer Res.*, **28**, 2349

VAN DUUREN, B.L., SIVAK, A., KATZ, C., SEIDMAN, I. and MELCHIONNE, S.M. (1975) *Cancer Res.*, **35**, 502
VAN DUUREN, B.L., SMITH, A.C. and MELCHIONNE, S.M. (1978) *Cancer Res.*, **38**, 865
WEBER, J. and HECKER, E. (1978) *Experientia,* **34**, 679
WEINSTEIN, A.B. (1981) *J. Supramolec. Struct. Cell Biochem.*, **17**, 99
WEINSTEIN, I.B. (1983) *Nature,* **302**, 750
WEINSTEIN, I.B., LEE, L.-S., FISHER, P.B., MUFSON, A. and YAMASAKI, H. (1979) In *Environmental Carcinogenesis*. Eds P. Emmelot and E. Kriek. pp. 265–285. Amsterdam: Elsevier/North-Holland Biomedical Press
WEINSTEIN, I.B., WIGLER, M., FISHER, P.B., SISSKIN, E. and PIETROPAOLO, C. (1978) In *Carcinogenesis*. Vol. 2: *Mechanisms of Tumor Promotion and Cocarcinogenesis*. Eds T.J. Slaga, A. Sivak and R.K. Boutwell. pp. 313–333. New York: Raven Press
WEINSTEIN, I.B., WIGLER, M. and PIETROPAOLO, C. (1977) In *Origins of Human Cancer*. Eds J.B. Watson and J.A. Winston. Cold Spring Harbor Conferences on Cell Proliferation. Vol. 4, pp. 751–752. Cold Spring Harbor Laboratory, Cold Spring Harbor, New York
WIGLER, M., DE FEO, D. and WEINSTEIN, I.B. (1978) *Cancer Res.*, **38**, 1434
WIGLER, M. and WEINSTEIN, I.B. (1976) *Nature,* **259**, 232
YAMASAKI, H., FIBACH, E., NUDEL, U., WEINSTEIN, I.B., RIFKIND, R.A. and MARKS, P.A. (1977) *Proc. Natl Acad. Sci. USA,* **74**, 3451
YAMASAKI, H., WEINSTEIN, I.B., FIBACH, E., RIFKIND, R.A. and MARKS, P.A. (1979) *Cancer Res.*, **39**, 1989
YUSPA, S.H., BEN, T., PATTERSON, E., MICHAEL, D., ELGIO, K. and HENNINGS, H. (1976) *Cancer Res.*, **36**, 4062

Chapter 7

Standard mutational theory of cancer and the impact of contingent advances in genetics

From what has been said already, it will be appreciated that a great deal is known about the initiating mechanisms of cellular transformation, but that the state of knowledge of subsequent biological events has not yet been developed to such an extent (Chapters 2–6). The regulation of mitosis, cell division, gene expression and differentiation, and the derangement of such regulating mechanisms, would seem to be incompletely understood. Thus, it is difficult to define the changes in the transformation of normal cells into tumour cells and the sequence of their occurrence. But, clearly, these changes involve a permanent heritable alteration in those properties that are due to the response of genotypic characters to the cellular environment, i.e. in 'phenotype'. Essentially, this amounts to a mutation, and cancer has for long been suspected to result from a single mutation or mutations.

Somatic cell mutation

The chromosomes were thought to be involved with malignant growth, soon after their discovery in 1887. Thus, Von Hansemann (1890) described in great detail, in a series of papers, the frequency of abnormal mitotic spindles and other mitotic abnormalities that occur in tumours. His suggestion that abnormal mitosis might be the cause of neoplasia was stressed by Boveri (1912, 1914), who postulated that malignancy was due to abnormal chromosome make-up of the tumour cell, following abnormal mitosis. This amounts to the 'chromosome theory of cancer', which was based on a parallelism between tumour cells and the double fertilization of sea-urchin eggs. Boveri's theory (1914) was slow to gain ground, as supporting evidence was not forthcoming because of unsatisfactory methodology, but, recently, a great deal of information has been obtained about normal cells and tumour cells. Chromosome anomalies have now been detected in many animal and human tumours, and their incidence would seem to favour Boveri's theory (Koller, 1960). In chronic myelogenous leukaemia, cells have been found with a chromosome which has undergone a slight deletion, viz. the so-called 'Philadelphia' chromosome (Nowell and Hungerford, 1960a,b; Tjio et al., 1966). Certain types of chromosome aberration have been found in other tumours (De Grouchy and de Nava, 1968). Monoclonal tumour development has been demonstrated for myoma of the uterus (Linder and Gartler, 1965), as well as for lymphoma, myeloma, chronic granulocytic leukaemia, multicentric liver and colon carcinoma (Beutler, Collins and Irwin, 1967; Fialkow, Gartler and Yoshida, 1967). Autosomal recessive diseases, Bloom's syndrome, Fanconi's anaemia and ataxia telangiectasia are associated with a high frequency of chromosome breakages and reunion, i.e. chromosome mutation, and patients suffering from these diseases are susceptible to an increased risk of developing leukaemia and several types of cancer (Hecht, 1966; Schroeder, 1972).

The possibility arises that chromosomal aberrations and the tissue specificity of tumour induction may be independent effects of chemical carcinogens. Thus, Röhrborn (1974) speculated that a carcinogen which induces cancer in one organ, might cause chromosomal aberrations in other tissues and, on the other hand, that an organotropic response to a chemical carcinogen may represent a later stage than the mutation/induction stage, possibly regulated by immunological processes and other factors. Mibelli's porokeratosis is an autosomal dominant trait, associated with malignant carcinomas. The patients' lymphocytes have normal chromosomes but fibroblasts, cultured from biopsies of areas with skin lesions, showed increased frequencies of chromosome gaps, breaks and reunions, whereas autopsies of unaffected skin areas did not usually show these chromosomal aberrations (Harnden, 1973; Taylor, Harnden and Fairburn, 1973). In this case, however, fibroblasts cannot be regarded as premalignant cells, as they do not participate directly in the development of the types of cancer that are concerned with this disease. Again, xeroderma pigmentosum is an autosomal recessive disease associated with skin neoplasia, but chromosomal aberrations are found in the cells only after exposure to u.v. light. Thus, these abnormal cells seem to have arisen from excessively rapid growth and other manifestations of malignancy (Koller, 1960), but they do not necessarily belong to the causative mechanism.

Boveri's theory is at any rate an important predecessor of the 'somatic cell (cells other than reproductive cells) mutation' theory of cancer (Bauer, 1928, 1949; Strong, 1949), which was enunciated to explain the irreversibility of neoplasia and the variety of human tumour types. The theory of somatic cell mutations infers that a subtle change or changes occur(s) to the genome, which may not be detectable morphologically, and which endow(s) the cell with new properties, whilst maintaining its cellular variability (Gause, 1966).

After it had been established that mutations in germ cells (reproductive cells) could be induced artificially in *Drosophila melanogaster* by X-rays (Muller, 1927) and chemical substances (Auerbach, Robson and Carr, 1947), it became feasible to study the correlation between mutagenesis in say *Drosophila* and carcinogenesis in mammals. Whilst a good correlation was found in early work (Auerbach, 1939; Tatum, 1947; Carr, 1948, 1950; Demerec, 1948; Latarjet, Buü-Hoi and Elias, 1950), there were some exceptions (Latarjet, 1948; Vogt, 1948; Berenblum and Shubik, 1949; Burdette, 1950; Burdette and Haddox, 1954; Fishbein, Flamm and Falk, 1970). It would probably have been quite unrealistic to have expected an absolute correlation, as mutagenic action might be supposed to be expressed in different ways, since some chemical substances behave as mutagens in some biological systems but not in other ones, and carcinogenic action does not appear to be an all-or-none phenomenon. Better correlations have been made, however, using sensitive *Salmonella typhimurium* strains modulated by mammalian liver microsomes in the Ames test (Ames and McCann, 1976; Bartsch, Malaveille and Montesano, 1976; Montesano and Bartsch, 1976; Purchase *et al.*, 1976, 1978; Davis *et al.*, 1980) (Chapter 2) and mammalian cells (Fox, 1975; Kuroki *et al.*, 1980).

Furthermore, mathematical analysis (Charles and Luce-Clausen, 1942; Iversen and Arley, 1950; Fisher and Hollomon, 1951; Nordling, 1953; De Waard, 1964) showed a consistency between these data but, of course, it did not prove that the theory of somatic cell mutations is correct.

The theory readily accounts for the irreversibility of neoplastic transformation and the variety of human tumour types, but, at the start, it was impossible, however, to devise an experimental system to test its validity. In fact, Haldane (1934, 1954) considered that the theory could neither be proved nor disproved, since it was impossible to test for mutation in somatic cells by crossing the supposed mutated cell with a normal cell and analysing the progeny. At that time, it was not feasible to hybridize somatic cells and to decode the DNA. Nevertheless, the theory of somatic cell mutations incorporates a great deal of the experimental evidence and inductive reasoning relating to chemical carcinogenesis, and it is universally true that all authentic chemical carcinogens are mutagens (but not necessarily vice versa).

In developing the theme of this chapter, it would now seem to be timely to try to bridge the gap between standard mutational theory and the resurgence of approaches to the study of the 'oncogenes' and the genetic redistribution (rearrangement of DNA) which can occur. The consideration of some models for carcinogenesis seems to be apposite.

Cancer models

Action of oncogenic viruses and chemical carcinogens

The possibility of such diverse agents causing cancer must be attributable to their effecting a change in the cell genome which induces a protumour alteration in cellular activity. This model would account for the genotypic change that is typified by:

(a) Irreversibility of neoplasia.
(b) Diversity of tumour type.
(c) The multiplicity of initiating chemical carcinogens.
(d) The apparent rarity of the carcinogenic event.
(e) The eventual pathological nature of the changes.

This model infers that:

(a) There ought to be some correlation between the capacity of a substance to cause germ mutations in the lower organisms and to induce tumours in mammals.
(b) Whilst mutation is very rapid, phenotypic expression parallels the long latent period of carcinogenesis.
(c) The incidence of multiple tumours might be expected to be greater for oncogenic viruses than chemical carcinogens, as only a small proportion of chemical mutations is likely to cause tumours.
(d) Neoplastic transformation ought to be inducible both by chemical carcinogens and by viruses *in vitro*.

All four points deserve comment. In the first place, there is a fair correlation between gene mutation and the tumours induced by a range of chemical substances, especially in the case of the ultimate carcinogens (Chapters 2, 3).

With regard to the second point, the rate of the initial transformation of a normal cell into a protumour cell has been found to be rapid both in the case of chemically induced skin cancer *in vivo* (Mottram, 1944; Gelboin, Klein and Bates, 1965) and in that of chemically (Chapter 3) and virally induced cancer *in vitro* (Manaker and Groupé, 1956; Temin and Rubin, 1958; Vogt and Dulbecco, 1960; Sachs and Medina, 1961; Koprowski *et al.*, 1962; Rapson and Kirschstein, 1962; Black and Rowe, 1963; McBride and Wilner, 1964; McAllister and Macpherson, 1967).

Thirdly, this argument seems to be equivocal, as multiple tumours of various type follow both polyoma virus infection and exposure to some chemical carcinogens, for example to 2AAF and various nitrosamines.

Fourthly, the transformation of normal cells into tumour cells *in vitro* can be implemented both by various viruses (Vogt and Dulbecco, 1960; Sachs and Medina, 1961) and by chemical carcinogens (Berwald and Sachs, 1965; Chen and Heidelberger, 1969).

The foregoing model has the further merit that it would serve also for the oncogenic RNA viruses, since they induce the cell to produce DNA proviruses which can be incorporated into the cellular DNA genome (Temin, 1971; Hill and Hillova, 1972; Karpas and Milstein, 1973). Production of DNA proviruses proceeds by reverse transcription, and the DNA proviruses would serve as templates for replication of RNA viruses (Temin, 1966; Spiegelman *et al.*, 1970). An RNA-directing polymerase, which was first extracted from the viruses *per se* (Baltimore, 1970; Temin and Mizutani, 1970), has been detected subsequently in normal uninfected cells (Scolnick *et al.*, 1971; Sarngadharan *et al.*, 1972).

This model is open to the criticism that the phenotypic expression of the genotypic change, which appears to take the form of a multistage process (Chapter 6), would necessitate additional factors.

Genetic control

Jacob and Monod (1961) suggested that differentiation might be regulated by the switching on or off of specific genes in response to an exogenous inducer or to an end-product of intermediary metabolism. Cancer might result through the (pathological) derangement of such a control mechanism (Pitot and Heidelberger, 1963). It is relevant that evidence had been found in the case of certain carcinogenic amino-azo dyes for the covalent binding of reactive intermediates to target-cell proteins (Miller and Miller, 1947; Heidelberger and Moldenhauer, 1956; Miller, 1970) as well as to appropriate nucleic acids (amongst others *see* Brookes and Lawley, 1964) (Chapter 3). After prolonged administration of the carcinogen, when hepatomas had begun to develop, the capacity of the hepatocytes for protein binding was lost, and it was inferred (Miller and Miller, 1953) that the protein(s) concerned had been deleted from the cell. These workers (Miller and Miller, 1953) considered that, by corollary, protein deletion was important to neoplastic transformation. Whence, protein biosynthesis would require (Jacob and Monod, 1961):

(*a*) Structural genes that code for mRNA (transcription), which directs the biosynthesis of specific proteins in the cytosol (translation).
(*b*) An operator which, in the depressed state, permits transcription of the structural genes.
(*c*) A regulator gene which represses the operator through combination.

These concepts were elaborated by Pitot and Heidelberger (1963).

In essence, derepression enabled dormant cellular genes to function by normal processes, whereas the induction of tumours was considered to involve pathological change. The fact that derepression produces additional activity implied expression at a higher level of differentiation, whereas the cancer process seemed to operate at a lower level. But, even were these criticisms waived, and were Pitot and Heidelberger's model (1963) assumed to fit the chemical carcinogenesis process, it would not account for viral oncogenesis.

The 'oncogenes'

Originally, this concept (Huebner and Todaro, 1969; Huebner, 1970) stemmed from the fact that:

(a) Contagion is rare and the vertical transmission of oncogenic viruses is common in animals.
(b) The most common form of vertical transmission, for example in murine leukaemia and mammary cancer, is associated with the C-type RNA virus particles, which bud through mammalian cell membranes.
(c) Such C-type RNA virus particles are widespread in vertebrate tissues.

The model demands that these C-type RNA viruses are potential causative agents of all forms of cancer. These virus particles would carry an indigenous source of genetic information for neoplasia, transmitted to them from an 'oncogene' of the cellular DNA genome, but they would require activation to endow them with new transforming capacity. Such activation might be represented by derepression (Culliton, 1972). Supporting experiments were described (Freeman et al., 1970, 1971; Huebner et al., 1972), where the combined action of an oncogenic virus and a chemical carcinogen resulted in the formation of tumours *in vitro*, which were not produced by either one of these agents alone. But, the fact that this synergism occurs under prescribed experimental conditions does not, in itself, provide convincing evidence for an all-embracing theory. Expressed in these terms, the paradigm seems to raise as many problems as it provides explanation for. Thus, it was difficult to account for the activation necessary for the derivation of the expression of oncogenic action, and the genetic information contained by C-type mutants was considered to be inconsistent with the variety of resulting tumours.

Nevertheless, a model that stresses the key importance of a cellular 'oncogene' (Todaro and Huebner, 1972; Commings, 1973) is crucial to modern theory. During carcinogenesis, the activation of a normally innocuous cellular DNA sequence (or gene) would afford such an 'oncogene' that is endowed with new transforming capacity, compared with the original gene. It is noteworthy that:

(a) The origin of the oncogenic (nucleotide) sequences would be endogenous, and it would not have been imposed externally, for example as a viral macromolecule, on the cellular genome.
(b) The DNA sequences, which encode transformation, would make a distinct unit that would be an allelomorph of a normal cellular gene (and each gene, for example of a mammalian cell, would occur as a genetically dominant allelic form and as a recessive one).

It follows that the transformation of normal cells into tumour cells would appear to require the activation of specific cellular genes, and not of large segments of the cellular DNA genome.

The 'oncogene'/proto-oncogene concept

The foregoing model anticipates the subject matter concerned with 'oncogenes' and proto-oncogenes. It is generally considered that the underlying ideas are best developed through description of the viral 'oncogenes'*. One class of 'oncogenes' and proto-oncogenes has been discovered from work on the retroviruses that cause cancer in some animals, and of which the genetic material is composed of RNA (and not DNA). The RNA is reverse transcribed into DNA through the viral infection of a cell. It ought to be explained that the RNA- or retro- viruses have been shown to bear a single gene, viz. an 'oncogene', which is responsible for cancer induction. The idea developed that such viral 'oncogenes' originated as mammalian proto-oncogenes, which were trapped, translated into RNA (and therefore without inserts) and transported or transduced by retroviruses which infect animal cells. Somehow or other these proto-oncogenes become 'oncogenes' after incorporation into the retrovirus genome and the transforming properties thus acquired are expressed when 'oncogenes' are inserted (through viral infection) into the mammalian genomes as intact viral RNA macromolecules.

The foregoing concept of the transformation of normal (mammalian) cellular genes or proto-oncogenes into 'oncogenes' by viral regulation is an extremely important one, as it is quite easy to understand that the carcinogenic process may involve, for example, gene mutations, amplification, transposition and rearrangement.

Up-to-date, 17 or so such cellular proto-oncogenes have been defined, and each of them is known from its association, as an active 'oncogene', with a particular retrovirus. Interestingly, there appeared to be two classes of normal proto-oncogenes and their 'oncogene' counterparts. One group (*see above*) was discovered by gene transfer or transfection, which detects essentially dominant (in the genetic sense) changes, and comprised those 'oncogenes' that arose from the mutation of proto-oncogenes (Blair *et al.*, 1981; Hayward, Neel and Astrin, 1981; Karess and Hanafusa, 1981). A second group had been found previously, and was made up of genes that had somehow become activated by retroviruses. These two groups are not mutually exclusive, however, as hybridization experiments had shown that some 'oncogenes' from human tumours were closely related, structurally and functionally, to those 'oncogenes', carried by several retroviruses which infected animals, for example rats. A human bladder carcinoma 'oncogene' was closely related to the 'oncogene' which is transduced by the Harvey sarcoma virus and trapped from the rat genome. This means that the same proto-oncogene is activated either by mutation in human subjects or by retroviral acquisition and regulation. Another proto-oncogene is activated in human subjects to produce human bladder, colon, lung and pancreas carcinomas as well as some human sarcoma or it is activated by incorporation into the Kirsten rat-sarcoma virus. These two cellular proto-oncogenes are themselves related evolutionarily. Another human 'oncogene', called *N-ras*, occurs in the native DNA of various leukaemias, a lymphoma, a neuroblastoma, a colon carcinoma as well as various sarcomas. Clearly, the presence of the foregoing *ras* 'oncogenes' in the native DNA of a variety of tumours suggests that activation of a particular cellular proto-oncogene is not the specific property of any single tissue. Thus, for example, the same gene,

---

*There is, however, nothing unique about this choice of material and, for example, the results of contemporaneous work with *Drosophila* were interpreted in terms of another class of 'oncogenes' and proto-oncogenes.

activated in any one of a number of tissues, would induce in each one of them a different type of tumour.

The rest of the narrative of this chapter is concerned with a more detailed development of some aspects of the 'oncogene'/proto-oncogene concept and the outcome as far as this has progressed.

It seems feasible that the activation of cellular 'oncogenes' by retroviruses might be brought about by increased dosage of a normal cellular protein to produce a phenotype, which is not realized at low level expression, and available experimental evidence (Hughes et al., 1979; Oppermann et al., 1979; Sefton. Hunter and Beemon, 1980; Coffin et al., 1981; Klein, 1981) seems to support this supposition. Accordingly, the virtually identical, cellular onc proteins, which are present in low concentration in normal cells, would not exert an oncogenic effect on cellular phenotype.

For the model which was used for transformation of normal cellular genes into 'oncogenes' by viral regulation to be tenable for the similar transformation by chemical carcinogens, an equivalent activation would have to be brought about through the rearrangement of blocs of normal cellular (nucleotide) sequences, following significant carcinogen interaction with DNA. The same genes would not necessarily be activated by chemical carcinogens in the new ideal model/theory as the ones that were expropriated and activated by retroviruses. This inductive reasoning underlines the creative work of Weinberg et al. (Shih et al., 1979, 1981; Shilo and Weinberg, 1981) in this subject area.

Again, gene transfer proved to be a useful investigational tool for tackling the problems concerned. According to the method of Graham and van der Eb (1973), DNA might be coprecipitated with $Ca_3(PO_4)_2$ and the crystals deposited on and assimilated by monolayers of cultured cells. By these means, a small proportion of the intact DNA that was applied was found to be taken up by the cells, its presence being expressed both in the recipient cells and in the progeny, i.e. in the descendant daughter cells. In this way, Shih et al. (1979) introduced 3-methylcholanthrene-transformed mouse-fibroblast DNA into normal, untransformed fibroblasts and transformed these recipient cells. The control experiment, involving DNA from untransformed donor cells, did not induce transformation in the recipient monolayer bed of cells. This evidence proved that the DNA of 3-methylcholanthrene-initiated cells was structurally different from that of the controls, and this has to do with phenotype, as the oncogenic information conveyed by DNA transfer is responsible for the transformation phenotype in the donor cell-line from which the DNA was prepared. Thus, in chemically transformed cells, modification of DNA occurs in those regions of the cellular DNA genome which elicit a transformation phenotype. A caveat must be entered to the effect that these experiments do not shed light on the mechanisms by which a mutagen that interacts with DNA induces the activation of cellular oncogenic (nucleotide) sequences.

Evidence (amongst others Shih et al., 1979, 1981; Krontiris and Cooper, 1981; Shilo and Weinberg, 1981) is beginning to accrue, however, which begins to suggest that the transforming genes, discussed in the foregoing narrative, may represent activated, possibly rearranged, forms of normal cellular (nucleotide) sequences, which may or may not be associated with retrovirus genomes.

The developing 'oncogene' story

The foregoing version of the 'oncogene' model, which stresses the importance of specific genes in the cellular DNA genome to initiation by reactive carcinogen intermediates, seems to mark another milestone in the elucidation of the mode of action of chemical carcinogens. But, in order to relate the 'oncogene' concept and related rearrangement of (nucleotide) sequences in the cellular genome, i.e. redistribution of genes, to the background of evidence on chemical carcinogenesis (Chapters 2–6), it would now appear to be germane to discuss various aspects of this and contingent ideas.

Transforming genes in some carcinogenic situations

Since the mammalian DNA genome may represent some $n \times 10^4$ genes, it is feasible that any one gene out of say $m \times 10^2$ genes may conceivably become an activated transforming gene in the previously described work with the 3-methylcholanthrene-transformed cells. Thus, any estimate of the number of such transforming genes would be valuable. It is therefore very interesting that in the case of four independently transformed (exposure to 3-methylcholanthrene) mouse-fibroblast cell-lines, the same cellular (nucleotide) sequence was activated each time to give a single transforming gene (Shilo and Weinberg, 1981). These workers (Shilo and Weinberg, 1981) treated each of the transforming DNAs with one of a series of restriction enzymes (i.e. site-specific endonucleases), and they then tested the reaction mixture for loss or retention of biological activity by gene transfer: as many as five different restriction enzymes were used for each of the four independently transformed mouse-fibroblast lines. Each cell-line gave an identical specific pattern, indicating that the same cellular (nucleotide) sequence was activated in each case to afford a single transforming gene. This approach therefore suggests that, despite the small number of independently transformed mouse fibroblasts which were employed, highly significant specificity attaches to individual 'oncogenes'.

Cell types responding in the transfection-focus assay

Before drawing a more general conclusion, however, it is worthwhile considering that fibroblastic elements pertain to sarcomas, and that what has been found for the active 'oncogenes' of the fibroblasts may not necessarily hold for the unrelated active 'oncogenes' of the non-fibroblastic transformants belonging to the carcinoma cells.

This argument seems to raise the matter of the scope and relevance of these experiments. In the transfection-focus assays used in this approach, cell-lines developed ideally from tumour cells are employed as donor cells and NIH3T3 mouse fibroblasts as recipients. The NIH3T3 mouse fibroblasts behave as very sensitive indicators of transforming genes from different sources (Krontiris and Cooper, 1981; Murray et al., 1981; Shih et al., 1981). Since human carcinoma and leukaemia DNAs respond in those transfection-focus assays, the action of these genes seems to be independent of tissue and species specificity. The fact that the DNAs of most types of mammalian tumours are inactive upon gene transfer, however, does appear to impose a rather serious limitation on this, otherwise attractive, experimental approach. It is uncertain whether unsuccessful transfer relates to current methodology or whether the (nucleotide) sequences of the non-transferable genes are, in fact, significantly different from the ones which have been considered hitherto.

The 'oncogenes' concerned

Whilst work on 3-methylcholanthrene-transformed mouse cells (*see above*) demonstrated the activation of a single 'oncogene' in four fibroblast transforming situations, that (Murray *et al.*, 1981) on the transforming genes of a human colon carcinoma, a bladder carcinoma and a myelogenous leukaemia cell-line revealed three different structures, thereby evoking three genes. In this case, analysis depended on the transfer of human genes through two cycles (of 'transfection') so that the transforming gene represents almost all of the human DNA in the final, transformed recipient cells. The outline of each was mapped, as human genes are embedded in complex segments of repetitive DNA sequences (Houck, Rinehart and Schmid, 1979). This type of analysis can be used in respect of other human transforming 'oncogenes' (Solomon and Goodfellow, 1983). The experimental evidence supports the conclusion (Murray *et al.*, 1981) that, in fact, three different genes had been studied.

Analogy between carcinogen-induced cellular 'oncogenes' and their viral counterparts

Data accruing about the carcinogen-activated 'oncogenes' suggest an analogy with virally activated 'oncogenes'. A first feature has to do with structural characteristics (of the sequences of the two groups). In both cases, the oncogenic sequences behave as if they were discrete blocs of (nucleotide) sequences which segregate on gene transfer as though they were, in fact, separate elements or genes. Virus- and carcinogen-induced 'oncogenes' each constitute groups of genes, but the size of these groups has not been determined. With regard to the virus-related 'oncogenes', there are at least eight members of this gene group (Coffin *et al.*, 1981). Secondly, the two groups of 'oncogenes' appear to originate from innocuous cellular (nucleotide) sequences, with no viral affinities, and they become subverted by carcinogen- or virus-mediated genetic rearrangements. This supposition is supported by the work on retrovirus *onc* genes.

These analogies suggest that the virus-associated *onc* genes would serve as an experimental model for carcinogen-initiated tumours with more difficult accessibility.

Activation of 'oncogenes'

To recapitulate, DNA-mediated gene-transfer methods facilitate the detection of dominant transforming genes ('oncogenes') in various human tumours (Cooper, 1982). Whilst only a few human tumour DNAs have been shown to be capable of transforming normal cells in the transection-focus assay, 'oncogenes' have been identified in representative tumours (Krontiris and Cooper, 1981; Lane, Sainten and Cooper, 1981, 1982; Murray *et al.*, 1981; Shih *et al.*, 1981).

Several (>10) different human 'oncogenes' have been identified, and one of these, which occurs in the T24 and EJ bladder carcinoma cell-lines, has been isolated by molecular cloning (Goldfarb *et al.*, 1982; Shih and Weinberg, 1982). Exploratory characterization showed this gene to be a small one (less than 4.6 kilobases), which has not been involved in major genetic rearrangement (Goldfarb *et al.*, 1982; Santos *et al.*, 1982; Shih and Weinberg, 1982). Analysis by retroviral transforming *onc* genes showed an internal fragment of the T24 'oncogene' to be closely related to the *onc* genes of Harvey and BALB murine sarcoma viruses (v-*has* and v-*bas*, respectively) (Der, Krontiris and Cooper, 1982; Parada *et al.*, 1982; Santos *et al.*, 1982). Furthermore, the characterization of human DNA sequences, homologous to v-*has* and v-*bas* showed that the normal c-*has*/c-*bas*-1 gene is in fact an allele of the T24 'oncogene' (Chang *et al.*, 1982b; Der, Krontiris and Cooper, 1982; Parada *et al.*, 1982; Santos *et al.*, 1982). These genes were indistinguishable from one another both by heteroduplex and by restriction enzyme analysis, despite their different biological properties (Der, Krontiris and Cooper, 1982; Parada *et al.*, 1982; Santos *et al.*, 1982). Hence, the nature of the genetic changes which elicited the activation of the T24 human bladder carcinoma 'oncogene' was investigated (Reddy *et al.*, 1982).

This work (Reddy *et al.*, 1982) showed that the genetic change which led to the activation of the 'oncogene' in T24 human bladder carcinoma cells, was brought about by a single point mutation of guanosine into thymidine, and that this alteration in sequence resulted in the incorporation of valine instead of glycine as the twelfth amino-acid residue of the T24 'oncogene'-encoded p21 protein. Thus, it looks as though a single qualitative difference, viz. the substitution of one amino acid for another, may be sufficient to confer transforming properties on the gene product of the T24 human bladder carcinoma 'oncogene' (Reddy *et al.*, 1982).

In this connection, Tsuchida, Ryder and Ohtsubo (1982) had investigated previously the nucleotide sequence of v-*kis*, the *onc* gene of Kirsten-MSV. Comparison of the first 37 amino acids in the deduced sequence of the Kirsten p21 protein with those of the T24 p21 protein showed only two differences, viz. serine in place of glycine in position 12 and glutamine in place of glutamic acid in position 37. So, it is feasible that changes in the glycine residue at position 12 may have activated also the c-*kis* genes. If this were the case, then several human carcinomas, known to contain the human c-*kis*-2 gene, may have been activated in the same way as the T24 'oncogene' is activated.

Unfortunately, it is uncertain how the possibility of what appears to be a single genetic change activating a human transforming gene relates to the multistage model which is accepted (Nordling, 1953; Armitage and Doll, 1957; Süss, Kinzel and Scribner, 1973; Berenblum, 1974; Whittemore, 1978) for tumour induction (Chapter 6). Thus, activation of the T24 'oncogenes' may represent a late and irreversible step in carcinogenesis and in this connection, the NIH3T3 mouse cells that were used to identify this 'oncogene' are considered to be preneoplastic, and thus not normal cells. The tumour source of the donor cells might also be instanced. On the other hand, the possibility that this 'oncogene' may operate at the initiation of the biological events leading to the induction of some tumours cannot be ruled out.

In a rather similar way, the transforming gene of a human lung carcinoma-derived cell line, Hs242, has been cloned and identified, in biologically active form, as c-*bas*/*has* (Yuasa *et al.*, 1983). The genetic lesion responsible for the transforming activity of this Hs242 'oncogene' has been localized as a point mutation in the second exon of its coding (nucleotide) sequence, whereby an adenine residue at position 150 was replaced by thymine at that site. This alteration results in the substitution of leucine for glutamine as the amino acid within codon 61 of the (translational) p21 protein encoded by this gene (Yuasa *et al.*, 1983). The site of activation of the Hs242 'oncogene' is accordingly, entirely different from that of T24 and EJ 'oncogenes'. (No changes at all were found in the first exon of its coding sequence, the region in which a point mutation proved responsible for the activation of those T24 and EJ bladder carcinoma 'oncogenes'.)

The identification of a new transforming c-*bas/has* allele in a human lung carcinoma-derived cell-line shows that *bas/has* may be activated in more than one sort of tissue.

It is extremely interesting that Chang *et al.* (1982a) have shown that c-*bas/has* can acquire transforming properties when its coding region is subjected to the influence of the strong promoter-sequence signals of a retroviral long terminal repetitive (nucleotide) unit. This finding would appear to imply that high levels of the ordinary, normal p21 gene product can also induce cell transformation. In the event, the work of Yuasa *et al.* (1983) indicates, however, that qualitative, rather than quantitative, alterations are probably the most common cause of the acquisition of transforming properties under natural conditions *in vivo*.

Proteins encoded by activated 'oncogenes'

'Oncogene' theory, and possibly in particular the work of Chang *et al.* (1982a), received a boost by the identification, for the first time, of an endogenous protein with known physiological effects on normal cells as the product of an 'oncogene'. Two groups of workers (Doolittle *et al.*, 1983; Waterfield *et al.*, 1983) have found independently that the *sis* 'oncogene' encodes a protein similar to or identical with the platelet-derived growth factor, PDGF. Waterfield *et al.* (1983) described that a continuous sequence of 90 amino-acid residues (of PDGF) is identical in every respect to the predicted sequence (Devare *et al.*, 1983) of a large region in $p^{28}sis$, the putative transforming protein of simian sarcoma virus. In addition, Doolittle *et al.* (1983) discovered independently the same correlation from a somewhat less extensive sequencing of PDGT. Both discoveries depended on a computerized protein-sequence data-base, which had been established by Doolittle (1981), at the University of California in San Diego. As the cellular homologue, c-*sis*, of the viral *sis* gene is in fact present in the human DNA genome as a unique gene (Dalla-Favera *et al.*, 1981), it is most probably the gene concerned for PDGF.

The problem of establishing continuous amino-acid sequences in PDGF was very difficult, as this growth factor contained several peptide chains linked by cystinyl residues and, in this respect, it resembled epidermal growth factor (EGF), but the cloning of EGF mRNA showed EGF to be derived from a much larger precursor polypeptide (Gray, Dull and Ulbrich, 1983) that may contain other active peptides. If c-*sis* were the gene for PDGF, as was likely to be the case, then the sequencing of PDGF component peptides would become a much easier structural problem to tackle (Waterfield *et al.*, 1983).

It seems that PDGF is released from α-granules of platelets in blood coagulation, and it is the principal polypeptide growth factor in serum. As fibroblastic and neuroglial cells express PDGF receptors, they are particularly sensitive to the mitogenic (induction of cell division) action of PDGF (Heldin, Westermark and Wasteson, 1981). On binding the growth factor, the PDGF receptor shows tyrosine-specific kinase activity (Ek *et al.*, 1982), in the same way that EGF does (Cohen, Carpenter and King, 1980) (*see* Chapter 6). This type of protein phosphorylation is reminiscent of the enzyme activity of the *src* 'oncogenes' (Hunter and Sefton, 1980). 'Oncogenes' like *src* and *abl* encode a growth factor *per se*. On the assumption that the same cell produces both the factor and the receptor, then an autocrine stimulation (Sporn and Todaro, 1980) of proliferation will occur. It may be relevant that the tumours, which have been found to express the cellular homologue of the *sis* gene, are sarcomas and gliomas (Eva, 1982).

The apparent identity of a protein, which possesses well-established physiological effects, with the translational product of an 'oncogene' is extremely important. Cellular elements, like such oncogene proteins, appear to be crucial to the cancer process, but just how such proteins function is unclear. The work of Doolittle *et al.* (1983) and Waterfield *et al.* (1983) clearly infers that they regulate the growth of cells, on the assumption that the normal protein encoded by a proto-oncogene regulates normal growth and the form encoded by the corresponding 'oncogene' leads eventually to tumour growth. Thus, the degree of involvement of these molecules in transforming the activity of nucleotide sequences in the cellular genome, i.e. in transformation, may provide clues to the disturbance in growth control in procancer cells. It would appear that oncogenic function links with the mitogenic cascades induced by growth factors.

Concluding remarks

On present evidence, it is uncertain where the possibility of a single genetic change activating a mammalian transforming gene fits the generally accepted multistage model for tumour induction by chemical carcinogens. There is, however, strong evidence that:

(a) In the case of T24 human bladder carcinoma cells, 'oncogene' activation is effected by a single point mutation of guanosine into thymine, which in sequence resulted in the misincorporation of valine (instead of glycine) in the encoded protein, and that this conferred transforming properties on the gene product of the particular 'oncogene'.

(b) In the case of human lung carcinoma Hs242 cells, 'oncogene' activation is localized as a point mutation of adenosine into thymidine, which in turn resulted in the misincorporation of leucine (instead of glutamine) in the encoded protein, and that this conferred transforming properties on the gene product of that 'oncogene'.

Despite the fact that in the related transfection-focus assays, the donor cells were of tumour origin and the recipient NIH3T3 mouse-carcinoma cells were preneoplastic, whereas at the start of other work on the initiation of cells in normal living mammals by carcinogens (Chapters 2–4), no tumorigenic implications had arisen, there is a marked analogy between the data relating to the activation of an 'oncogene' (*see* (a) and (b)) and those concerning the interaction of reactive carcinogen intermediates with the cellular DNA genome. Thus, in the latter case, for example with vinyl chloride, imidazo cyclization of dA, dC and dG *in vivo* led to misincorporation of dG in poly(dA–dT) opposite dA *in vitro* and of dA or dT in poly(dC–dG) opposite dC, and to a lesser extent opposite dG, which would be consistent with the respective transversions:

(dA–dT) → (dC–dG) and (dC–dG) → (dA–dT)

by etheno-dA, etheno-dC and etheno-dG, which concur with the established base-pair substitution mutations for this carcinogen. These mutations would incur analogous changes in the corresponding translational (encoded) protein(s). Such findings may tentatively suggest that 'oncogene' activation, in the manner described, may relate to an early biological event in the transformation of normal cells into tumour cells by chemical carcinogens. In which case, the genetic approach stresses selection under natural conditions, by reactive carcinogen intermediates, from amongst whole segments of the cellular DNA genome of an innocuous gene and its activation into a transforming 'oncogene' *in vivo*.

Recent work (Doolittle *et al.*, 1983; Waterfield *et al.*, 1983) on naturally occurring encoded proteins in serum may evoke the possibility of 'oncogene' activation by dosimetry (Chang *et al.*, 1982a).

Natural carcinogenesis seems to be a multistage process (Chapter 6), and evidence for this comes from epidemiology. Thus, for example, the relationship between the incidence of lung cancer and the frequency and duration of cigarette smoking (Chapter 1) might be cited, as well as the conclusion of numerous laboratory experiments which showed that tumour induction resulted from several, apparently independent, rate-limiting steps (Chapter 6). It is feasible that provision of an active 'oncogene', whether through the activation of a normal cellular gene through rearrangement or mutation or by viral infection, presumably corresponds to only one of a sequence of steps. The 'oncogene' step is an entirely necessary stage, but normal cells have to undergo more than one independent alteration before they become *bona fide* tumour cells.

Side by side with the conspicuous advances made by Doolittle *et al.* (1983) and Waterfield *et al.* (1983), it is salutary to recall that, in the transfection-focus type of assay, many tumour types, irrespective of whether they are naturally occurring or whether they are produced by chemical carcinogens or X-rays, do not yield DNA that is oncogenic. Gene transfer necessarily relates to dominant changes, in the genetic sense. Consequently, this method will detect only 'oncogenes' which provide those specific products that the particular recipient cells require for their transformation. In addition, of course, transforming genes must not be too large to be capable of transfer intact.

In some tumours, for example in a Burkitt's lymphoma, two 'oncogenes' have been found which need to be activated, and such a finding may suggest that a requirement for the activation of more than one discrete 'oncogene' would be consistent with the multistage nature of carcinogenesis. Each 'oncogene' may elicit a different alteration within the cell and, taken collectively, these may confer important aspects of tumour phenotype.

What appears to have happened is that the different experimental approaches to chemical carcinogenesis now seem to be converging. Recent findings (this chapter) at the genetic level are consistent with the data resulting from epidemiological survey and analysis (*see* Chapter 1), and from the chemical/biochemical investigation of cellular transformation (Chapters 2–6).

Bibliography and references

AMES, B.N. and McCANN, J. (1976) In *Screening Tests in Chemical Carcinogenesis*. International Agency for Research on Cancer/WHO, Scientific Publications, no. 12, pp. 493–519. Lyon, France: IARC
ARMITAGE, P. and DOLL, R. (1957) *Br. J. Cancer,* **11**, 161
AUERBACH, C. (1939) *Proc. Intern. Congr. Genetics* 7th, p. 51
AUERBACH, C., ROBSON, J.M. and CARR, J.G. (1947) *Science,* **105**, 243
BALTIMORE, D. (1970) *Nature,* **226**, 1209
BARTSCH, H., MALAVEILLE, C. and MONTESANO, R. (1976) In *Screening Tests in Chemical Carcinogenesis*. International Agency for Research on Cancer/WHO, Scientific Publications, no. 12, pp. 467–491. Lyon, France: IARC
BAUER, K.H. (1928) *Mutationstheorie der Geschwulst-Entstehung*. Berlin: Julius Springer
BAUER, K.H. (1949) *Das Krebsproblem*. Berlin: Julius Springer

BERENBLUM, I. (1974) *Carcinogenesis as a Biological Problem.* pp. 43–49, 119–129. Amsterdam: North-Holland Publishing Company
BERENBLUM, I. and SHUBIK, P. (1949) *Br. J. Cancer,* **3**, 109
BERWALD, Y. and SACHS, L. (1965) *J. Natl Cancer Inst.,* **35**, 671
BEUTLER, E., COLLINS, Z. and IRWIN, L.E. (1967) *N. Engl. J. Med.,* **276**, 389
BLACK, P.H. and ROWE, W.P. (1963) *Proc. Soc. Exp. Biol. Med.,* **114**, 721
BLAIR, D.G., OSKARSSON, M., WOOD, T.G., McCLEMMENTS, W.L., FISCHINGER, P.J. and VAN DE WOUDE, G.C. (1981) *Science,* **212**, 941
BOVERI, T. (1912) Beitrag zum Studium des Chromatin in den Epithelzellen der Carcinome. *Beitr. Pathol. Anat.,* **14**, 249
BOVERI, T. (1914) *Zur Frage der Entstehung Maligner Tumoren.* Jena: Gustav Fischer
BROOKES, P. and LAWLEY, P.D. (1964) *Nature,* **202**, 781
BURDETTE, W.J. (1950) *Science,* **112**, 303
BURDETTE, W.J. and HADDOX, C.H. (1954) *Cancer Res.,* **14**, 167
CARR, J.G. (1948) *Br. J. Cancer,* **2**, 132
CARR, J.G. (1950) *Biochem. Soc. Symp.,* **4**, 25
CHANG, E.H., FURTH, M.E., SCOLNICK, E.M. and LOWY, D.R. (1982a) *Nature,* **297**, 479
CHANG, E.H., GONDA, M.A., ELLIS, R.W., SCOLNICK, E.M. and LOWY, D.R. (1982b) *Proc. Natl Acad. Sci. USA,* **79**, 4848
CHARLES, D.R. and LUCE-CLAUSEN, E.M. (1942) *Cancer Res.,* **2**, 261
CHEN, T.T. and HEIDELBERGER, C. (1969) *Int. J. Cancer,* **4**, 166
COFFIN, J.M., VARMUS, H.E., BISHOP, J.M., ESSEX, M., HARDY, W.D., MARTIN, G.S. *et al.* (1981) *J. Virol.,* **40**, 953
COHEN, S., CARPENTER, G. and KING, L. (1980) *J. Biol. Chem.,* **255**, 4834
COMMINGS, D.E. (1973) *Proc. Natl Acad. Sci. USA,* **70**, 3324
COOPER, G.M. (1982) *Science,* **217**, 801
CULLITON, B.J. (1972) *Science,* **177**, 44
DALLA FAVERA, R., GELMANN, E.P., GALLO, R.C. and WONG-STAAL, F. (1981) *Nature,* **292**, 31
DAVIS, A., DEVORET, R., GREEN, M., HOFNUNG, M., KAWACHI, T., MATSUSHIMA, T. *et al.* (1980) Report on Mutagenesis Assays with Bacteria. In *International Agency for Research on Cancer Monographs on the Evaluation of the Carcinogenic Risk of Chemicals to Humans,* Supplement 2, pp. 85–106. Lyon, France: IARC
DE GROUCHY, J. and DE NAVA, C. (1968) *Ann. Intern. Med.,* **69**, 381
DE WAARD, R.H. (1964) *Int. J. Radiat. Biol.,* **8**, 381
DEMEREC, M. (1948) *Br. J. Cancer,* **2**, 114
DER, C.J., KRONTIRIS, T.G. and COOPER, G.M. (1982) *Proc. Natl Acad. Sci. USA,* **79**, 3637
DEVARE, S.G., REDDY, P.E., LAW, P.D., ROBBINS, K. and AARONSON, S.A. (1983) *Proc. Natl Acad. Sci. USA,* **80**, 731
DOOLITTLE, R.F. (1981) *Science,* **214**, 149
DOOLITTLE, R.F., HUNKAPILLER, M.W., HOOD, L.E., DEVARE, S.G., ROBBINS, K.C., AARONSON, S.A. *et al.* (1983) *Science,* **221**, 275
EK, B., WESTERMARK, B., WASTESON, Å. and HELDIN, C.-H. (1982) *Nature,* **295**, 419
EVA, A. (1982) *Nature,* **295**, 116
FIALKOW, P.S., GARTLER, S.M. and YOSHIDA, A. (1967) *Proc. Natl Acad. Sci. USA,* **58**, 1468
FISHBEIN, L., FLAMM, W.G. and FALK, H.L. (1970) *Chemical Mutagens.* New York: Academic Press
FISHER, J.C. and HOLLOMON, J.H. (1951) *Cancer,* **4**, 916
FOX, M. (1975) *Mutat. Res.,* **29**, 449
FREEMAN, A.E., PRICE, P.J., IGEL, H.J., YOUNG, J.C., MARYAK, J.M. and HUEBNER, R.J. (1970) *J. Natl Cancer Inst.,* **44**, 65
FREEMAN, A.E., PRICE, P.J., BRYAN, R.J., GORDON, R.J., GILDEN, R.V., KELLOFF, G.J. *et al.* (1971) *Proc. Natl Acad. Sci. USA,* **68**, 445
GAUSE, G.F. (1966) In *Microbiological Models of Cancer Cells.* Chap. 1. Amsterdam: North-Holland
GELBOIN, H.V., KLEIN, M. and BATES, R.R. (1965) *Proc. Natl Acad. Sci. USA,* **53**, 1353
GOLDFARB, M., SHIMIZU, K., PERUCHO, M. and WIGLER, M. (1982) *Nature,* **296**, 404
GRAHAM, F.L. and VAN DER EB, A.J. (1973) *Virology,* **52**, 456
GRAY, A., DULL, T.J. and ULBRICH, A. (1983) *Nature,* **303**, 722
HALDANE, J.B.S. (1934) *J. Pathol. Bacteriol.,* **38**, 507
HALDANE, J.B.S. (1954) *The Biochemistry of Genetics.* pp. 100–110. London: George Allen and Unwin
HARNDEN, D.G. (1973) *Ataxia-telangiectasia Mibelli.* Dr. phil. dissertation, Heidelberg
HAYWARD, W.S., NEEL, B.G. and ASTRIN, S.M. (1981) *Nature,* **290**, 475
HECHT, F. (1966) *Lancet,* **ii**, 1193

HEIDELBERGER, C. and MOLDENHAUER, M.G. (1956) *Cancer Res.*, **16**, 442
HELDIN, C.-H., WESTERMARK, B. and WASTESON, Å. (1981) *Proc. Natl Acad. Sci. USA*, **78**, 3664
HILL, M. and HILLOVA, J. (1972) *Nat. New Biol.*, **237**, 35
HOUCK, C.M., RINEHART, F.P. and SCHMID, C.W. (1979) *J. Mol. Biol.*, **132**, 289
HUEBNER, R.J. (1970) In *Comparative Leukaemia Research*. Ed. R.M. Dutcher. p. 22. Basel: S. Karger
HUEBNER, R.J., FREEMAN, A.E., WHITMIRE, C.E., PRICE, P.J., RHIM, J.S., KELLOFF, G.J. et al. (1972) In *Environment and Cancer*. p. 295. Baltimore, Maryland: Williams and Wilkins Company
HUEBNER, R.J. and TODARO, G.J. (1969) *Proc. Natl Acad. Sci. USA*, **64**, 1087
HUGHES, S.H., PAYVAR, F., SPECTOR, D., SCHIMKE, R.T., ROBINSON, H.L., PAYNE, G.S. et al. (1979) *Cell*, **18**, 347
HUNTER, T. and SEFTON, B.M. (1980) *Proc. Natl Acad. Sci. USA*, **77**, 1311
IVERSEN, S. and ARLEY, N. (1950) *Acta Pathol. Microbiol. Scand.*, **27**, 773
JACOB, F. and MONOD, J. (1961) *Cold Spring Harb. Symp. Quant. Biol.*, **26**, 193
KARESS, R.E. and HANAFUSA, H. (1981) *Cell*, **24**, 155
KARESS, R.E., HAYWARD, W.S. and HANAFUSA, H. (1979) *Proc. Natl Acad. Sci. USA*, **76**, 3154
KARPAS, A. and MILSTEIN, C. (1973) *Eur. J. Cancer*, **9**, 295
KLEIN, G. (1981) *Nature*, **294**, 313
KOLLER, P.C. (1960) Chromosome behaviour in tumours: Readjustment to Boveri's theory. In *Cell Physiology and Neoplasia*. pp. 9–37. Austin, Texas: University of Texas Press
KOPROWSKY, H., PONTEN, J.A., JENSEN, F., RAVDIN, R.G., MOORHEAD, P. and SAKSELA, E. (1962) *J. Cell. Comp. Physiol.*, **59**, 281
KRONTIRIS, T. and COOPER, G.M. (1981) *Proc. Natl Acad. Sci. USA*, **78**, 1181
KUROKI, T., ABBONDONDOLO, A., DREVON, C., HUBERMAN, E. and LAVAL, F. (1980) Report on Mutagenesis Assays with Mammalian Cells. In *International Agency for Research on Cancer Monographs on the Evaluation of the Carcinogenic Risk of Chemicals to Humans*, Supplement 2, pp. 107–133. Lyon, France: IARC
LANE, M.A., SAINTEN, A. and COOPER, G.M. (1981) *Proc. Natl Acad. Sci. USA*, **78**, 1181
LANE, M.A., SAINTEN, A. and COOPER, G.M. (1982) *Cell*, **28**, 873
LATARJET, R. (1948) *C.R. Séances Soc. Biol.*, **142**, 453
LATARJET, R., BUÜ-HOI, N.P. and ELIAS, C.A. (1950) *Pubbl. Staz. zool Napoli*, Suppl. **22**, 78
LINDER, D. and GARTLER, S.M. (1965) *Science*, **150**, 67
McALLISTER, R.M. and MACPHERSON, E. (1967) *J. Gen. Virol.*, **2**, 555
McBRIDE, W.D. and WILNER, A. (1964) *Proc. Soc. Exp. Biol. Med.*, **115**, 870
MANAKER, R.A. and GROUPÉ, V. (1956) *Virology*, **2**, 838
MILLER, J.A. (1970) *Cancer Res.*, **30**, 559
MILLER, E.C. and MILLER, J.A. (1947) *Cancer Res.*, **7**, 468
MILLER, J.A. and MILLER, E.C. (1953) *Adv. Cancer Res.*, **1**, 339
MONTESANO, R. and BARTSCH, H. (1976) *Mutat. Res.*, **32**, 179
MOTTRAM, J.C. (1944) *J. Pathol. Bacteriol.*, **56**, 391
MULLER, H.I. (1927) *Science*, **66**, 84
MURRAY, M., SHILO, B., SHIH, C., CONNING, D., HSU, H.W. and WEINBERG, R.A. (1981) *Cell*, **25**, 355
NORDLING, C.O. (1953) *Br. J. Cancer*, **7**, 68
NOWELL, P.C. and HUNGERFORD, D.A. (1960a) *J. Natl Cancer Inst.*, **25**, 85
NOWELL, P.C. and HUNGERFORD, D.A. (1960b) *Science*, **132**, 1497
OPPERMANN, H., LEVINSON, A., VARMUS, H., LEVINTOV, L. and BISHOP, J.M. (1979) *Proc. Natl Acad. Sci. USA*, **76**, 1804
PARADA, L.F., TABIN, C.J., SHIH, C. and WEINBERG, R.A. (1982) *Nature*, **297**, 474
PITOT, H.C. and HEIDELBERGER, C. (1963) *Cancer Res.*, **23**, 1694
PURCHASE, I.F.H., LONGSTAFF, E., ASHBY, J., STYLES, J.A., ANDERSON, D., LEFÈVRE, P.A. et al. (1976) *Nature*, **264**, 624
PURCHASE, I.F.H., LONGSTAFF, E., ASHBY, J., STYLES, J.A., ANDERSON, D., LEFÈVRE, P.A. et al. (1978) *Br. J. Cancer*, **37**, 873
RAPSON, A.S. and KIRSCHSTEIN, R.L. (1962) *Proc. Soc. Exp. Biol. Med.*, **11**, 323
REDDY, P.E., REYNOLDS, R.K., SANTOS, E. and BARBACID, M. (1982) *Nature*, **300**, 149
RÖHRBORN, G. (1974) In *Chemical Carcinogenesis Essays*. International Agency for Research on Cancer Scientific Publications, no. 10, pp. 213–219. Lyon, France: IARC
SACHS, L. and MEDINA, D. (1961) *Nature*, **189**, 457
SANTOS, E., TRONICK, S.R., AARONSON, S.A., PULCIANI, S. and BARBACID, M. (1982) *Nature*, **298**, 343
SARNGADHARAN, M.G., SARIN, P.S., REITZ, M.S. and GALLO, R.C. (1972) *Nat. New Biol.*, **240**, 67
SCHROEDER, T.M. (1972) *Forschungsber. Med.*, **16**, 603
SCOLNICK, E.M., AARONSON, S.A., TODARO, G.J. and PARKS, W.P. (1971) *Nature*, **229**, 318

SEFTON, B.M., HUNTER, T. and BEEMON, K. (1980) *Proc. Natl Acad. Sci. USA,* **77**, 2059
SHIH, C., PADHY, L.C., MURRAY, M. and WEINBERG, R.A. (1981) *Nature,* **290**, 261
SHIH, C., SHILO, B., GOLDFARB, M.P., DANNENBERG, A. and WEINBERG, R.A. (1979) *Proc. Natl Acad. Sci. USA,* **76**, 5714
SHIH, C. and WEINBERG, R.A. (1982) *Cell,* **29**, 161
SHILO, B. and WEINBERG, R.A. (1981) *Nature,* **289**, 607
SOLOMON, E. and GOODFELLOW, P. (1983) *Nature,* **306**, 223
SPEIGELMAN, S., BURNY, A., DAS, M.R., KEYDAR, J., SCHLOM, J., TRAVNICEK, M. *et al.* (1970) *Nature,* **227**, 563
SPORN, M.B. and TODARO, G.J. (1980) *N. Engl. J. Med.,* **303**, 878
STRONG, L.C. (1949) *Yale J. Biol. Med.,* **21**, 293
SÜSS, R., KINZEL, V. and SCRIBNER, J.D. (1973) *Cancer: Experiments and Concepts.* pp. 53–63. New York: Springer-Verlag
TATUM, E.L. (1947) *Ann. N.Y. Acad. Sci.,* **49**, 87
TAYLOR, A.M.R., HARNDEN, D.G. and FAIRBURN, E.A. (1973) *J. Natl Cancer Inst.,* **51**, 371
TEMIN, H.M. (1966) *Cancer Res.,* **26**, 212
TEMIN, H.M. (1971) *J. Natl Cancer Inst.,* **46**, iii
TEMIN, H.M. and MITZUTANI, S. (1970) *Nature,* **226**, 1211
TEMIN, H.M. and RUBIN, H. (1958) *Virology,* **6**, 669
TJIO, J.H., CARBONE, P.P., WHANG, J. and FREI, E. (1966) *J. Natl Cancer Inst.,* **36**, 567
TODARO, G.J. and HUEBNER, R.J. (1972) *Proc. Natl Acad. Sci. USA,* **69**, 1009
TSUCHIDA, N., RYDER, T. and OHTSUBO, E. (1982) *Science,* **217**, 937
VOGT, M. (1948) *Experientia,* **4**, 68
VOGT, M. and DULBECCO, R. (1960) *Proc. Natl Acad. Sci. USA,* **46**, 365
VON HANSEMANN, D. (1890) *Virchows Arch. Pathol. Anat. Physiol. Klin. Med.,* **119**, 299
WATERFIELD, M.D., SCRACE, G.T., WHITTLE, N., STROOBANT, P., JOHNSSON, A., WASTESON, A. *et al.* (1983) *Nature,* **304**, 35
WEINSTEIN, I.B. (1983) *Nature,* **302**, 750
WHITTEMORE, A.S. (1978) *Adv. Cancer Res.,* **27**, 55
YUASA, Y., SRIVASTAVA, S.K., DUNN, C.Y., RHIM, J.S., REDDY, P.E. and AARONSON, S.A. (1983) *Nature,* **303**, 775

Index

Acetaldehyde, bromo-,
  carcinogenicity, 31
  covalent binding to DNA, 56–58
  metabolite,
    of 1,2-dibromoethane, 31
    of vinyl bromide, 30
—, chloro-,
  carcinogenicity, 30
  metabolite,
    of 1,2-dichloroethane, 31
    of vinyl chloride, 30
Acetamide, *N*-acetoxy-*N*-stilben-4-yl-,
  carcinogenicity,
    mechanism for, 49–52
—, *N*-deoxyguanosin-8-yl-*N*-fluoren-2-yl,
  carcinogenicity and, 47–50, 79
—, *N*-[3-(deoxyguanosin-N^2-yl)fluoren-2-yl]-,
  carcinogenicity and, 47–50, 79
—, *N*-fluoren-2-yl,
  carcinogenicity, 15, 86–87, 106
    mechanism for, 18–20
  N-sulphate salt,
    carcinogenicity, 18–20
—, 2-fluorenyl-,
  N-hydroxylation product,
    chemical activation and carcinogenicity, 16, 17–20, 37, 86–87
Aflatoxin,
  carcinogenicity, 6
—, B_1,
  as carcinogen,
    chemical activation, 33–34
    DNA synthesis and mutagenesis/carcinogenesis, 78
    inhibition of tumour induction, 88
    reaction with DNA, 60
—, G_1,
  as carcinogen,
    chemical activation, 34
    reaction with DNA, 60–61
Alkylation,
  in DNA synthesis,
    carcinogenesis and, 47–64

Alkylation (*cont.*)
  in DNA synthesis (*cont.*)
    effect on synthesis of inter-related macromolecules, 79–82
    inhibition of, 85–95
    miscoding during, 73–79
    promotion of subthreshold dose, 100–112
    repair of biochemical lesions formed, 68–72
Amino-azo dyes,
  carcinogenicity, 2–3
    inhibition by riboflavin, 90–91
    mechanism, 21–24
    protein binding, 18–19, 50–54
Aniline,
  bladder cancer, 2
—, 2,4,5-trimethyl-,
  mutagen and carcinogen from Ponceau 3R, 23
Aroclors, *see* Biphenyls, polychlorinated
Aromatic amines,
  carcinogenicity, 2–3, 14
    inhibition of, 86–87
    mechanism for, 47–54, 79
  mutagenicity, 16
  reactive metabolites, 15–16, 17–21, 36–37
Arylhydroxylamines, 17–21, 36–37
Asbestosis and carcinogenesis, 3–4
Azo-benzene, *p*-amino-,
  as carcinogen, 23–24
—, *p*-dimethylamino-,
  as carcinogen, 15, 23–24
  protein binding, 50–54
—, *p*-methylamino-,
  as carcinogen, 23–24
  mechanism, 47–48
  protein binding, 18–19, 50–54
Azotoluene, *o*-amino-,
  as carcinogen, 23–24

Benz[a]anthracene, 7-bromoethyl-,
  persistence of nucleoside analogues in target-organ, DNA, RNA etc., 72

Benz[a]anthracene, (cont.)
—, 7,12-dimethyl-,
  carcinogenicity,
    inhibition of induced tumours in animals, 87–89
    initiator of two-stage skin-system for carcinogenesis, 102, 109
    reactive benzilic ester metabolites, 33
Benzene,
  as leukaemogen, 5–6
Benzidine,
  carcinogen from amino-azo dyes, 22–23
  carcinogenicity, 2
    reactive metabolites, 37
    transport form, 37
—, 3,3'-dimethyl-,
  carcinogen from amino-azo dyes, 23
Benzo[a]pyrene,
  carcinogenicity, 15
    effect of modified DNA on transcription, 81
    inhibition of tumour induction, 87–89
    initiator of two-stage skin-system for carcinogenesis, 101
    persistence of covalent binding in target-organ DNA, RNA etc., 72
    reaction with DNA, 61–64
    reactive epoxide metabolites, 31–33
BHA, see Phenol, 2- and 3-tert-butyl-4-methoxy-
BHBN, see Nitrosamine, N-n-butyl-N-(4-hydroxybutyl)-
BHT, see Toluene, 4-hydroxy-3,5-di-tert-butyl-
Bile acids and salts,
  as promoters, 104
Biphenyl, 4-amino-,
  as human and animal carcinogen, 3
  reactive metabolite, 18
  transport form, 21
—, 4-amino-4'-fluoro-,
  reaction with DNA,
    carcinogenesis and, 47–49
—, N-deoxyguanosin-8-yl-4-acetylamino-, 4'-fluoro-,
  carcinogenesis and, 48
—, N-deoxyguanosin-8-yl-4-amino-4'-fluoro-,
  carcinogenesis and, 48
—, polychloro-,
  as inhibitors of tumour induction, 86

Cadmium,
  as carcinogen,
    effect on RNA synthesis, 81
    mechanism of action, 29
Cancer,
  as a systematic disease, 1–2, 7–11, 101–102, 113–115
Cancer genes, 117
  genetic control, 116–117
  gene transformation, 117, 119, 124–125
  'oncogene'/proto-oncogene concept, 118–119
    chemical carcinogens and, 119–125

Carcinogenesis,
  mechanisms of biological significance, 67–84
Carcinogenic potency in animals, 67
Carcinogenicity,
  chemical reactivity and, 47–48, 50, 54–56, 58, 60, 64
  industrial processes and, 2–4, 5–6, 7, 14–15
  matching tissue specificities, 36–38
    and spill-over model for mutagenicity/carcinogenicity, 38–41
  mechanisms in perspective, 67–112
  metabolism and, 17–36
Carcinogens,
  alkylating,
    mechanisms of, 47–64
  ethylating,
    mechanisms of action, 54–55
  industrial, 50, 53, 56–59, 61–62
  metals,
    DNA-repair and, 71
    mechanism of action, 56
  methylating,
    direct acting, 24–26
    mechanisms of reaction, 54–55
  naturally occurring,
    mechanisms of, 60–61, 63–64
Cellular aspects,
  in carcinogenesis, 101–102, 105–109, 113–117
Chemical carcinogenesis,
  mechanisms,
    summary and significance, 64–84
  as multistage process,
    bladder system, 105
    liver system, 105–106
    skin system, 101–102
Chloral,
  metabolite of trichloroethylene, 38–39
Chromium,
  as carcinogen,
    mechanism of action, 29
    miscoding induced in directed DNA biosynthesis, 77
  as mutagen, 16–77
Chrysoidine,
  as carcinogen, 23
Croton oil, see Phorbol esters
Cyanate, sodium,
  as inhibitor of polycyclic aromatic hydrocarbon carcinogenesis, 88
Cycasin,
  as carcinogen,
    reaction with DNA, 34–35
Cyclamate,
  as promoter, 104–105
Cyclophosphamide,
  as promoter, 105
Cysteamine,
  as inhibitor of DMN-tumours, 94
Cysteine, N-acetyl-S-(2-hydroxyethyl)-,
  metabolite of vinyl chloride, 39

… Index 131

Cysteine, (cont.)
—, S-(carboxymethyl)-,
  metabolite of vinyl chloride, 39
  metabolite of vinylidene chloride, 93

DEN, see Nitrosamine, N,N-diethyl-
Diazonium ions, ethyl-,
  derived from diethylnitrosamine,
    cyclic mechanism, 25–26
  derived from direct-acting N-ethyl-N-
    nitrosourea etc., 24–26
  mechanism of action, 54–55
—, methyl-,
  derived from cycasin,
    cyclic mechanism, 34–35
  derived from 1,1- and 1,2-dimethylhydrazines,
    cyclic mechanisms, 26–27
  derived from dimethylnitrosamine,
    cyclic mechanism, 25–26
  derived from direct-acting N-methyl-N-
    nitrosourea, N-methyl-N'-nitro-N-
    nitrosoguanidine etc., 24–25
  derived from triazenes,
    cyclic mechanism, 28–29
  mechanism of action, 54–55
Dichlorvos,
  mutagenicity and carcinogenicity,
    spill-over model for metabolism, 39–40
Direct Black 38,
  as carcinogen, 22–23
Direct Blue 6,
  as carcinogen, 22–23
Direct Brown 95,
  as carcinogen, 22–23
Disulphiram,
  as inhibitor of tumorigenesis, 88–90
DMN, see Nitrosamine, N,N-dimethyl-
DMPT, see Triazene, 3,3-dimethyl-1-phenyl
DNA-repair,
  O^6-alkylguanine and,
    in carcinogenesis, 68–72
DNA-synthesis,
  O^4-alkylthymine, O^4-alkyluracil and O^6-
    alkylguanine in carcinogenesis and, 73–79
  rate of synthesis,
    and inter-relationship with that of other
      macromolecules, 79–82
Druckrey–Küpfmüller relationship, 67

EMS, see Ethyl methane sulphonate
Endonuclease excision,
  and DNA-repair, 70–72, 95–97
ENNG, see Guanidine, N-ethyl-N'-nitro-N-
  nitroso-
ENU, see Urea, N-ethyl-N-nitroso-
Epidemiological data, 2–7, 125
Epoxide hydratase, 31–34, 38–39, 87–88
Ethane, 1,2-dibromo-,
  carcinogenicity,
    mechanism for, 31

Ethane, (cont.)
—, 1,2-dichloro-,
  carcinogenicity,
    mechanism for, 30, 56–58, 77–78
Ethylene oxide, chloro-,
  metabolite of vinyl chloride, 30
  reaction with DNA, 56–58
  rearrangement and reaction with DNA, 30,
    56–58
—, 1,1-dichloro-,
  metabolite of vinylidene chloride,
    rearrangement to form chloroacetyl chloride,
      93–94
—, 1,1,2-trichloro-,
  metabolite of 1,1,2-trichloroethylene,
    rearrangements in vitro and in vivo, 38–39
Ethylene, 1,1,2-trichloro-,
  metabolism,
    and carcinogenicity, spill-over model, 38–39
Ethyl methane sulphonate,
  direct-acting carcinogen, 9

Glutathione,
  protective pole against tumour induction, 93–94
Glutathione S-epoxide transferase, 30, 38, 93
Glutathione S-transferase-1,1, 53
Glycerol, diacetyl,
  as endogenous tumour promoter, 107
Glycidaldehyde,
  carcinogenicity,
    mechanism for, 58–59
  reaction with deoxyguanosine,
    carcinogenicity and, 59
Glycidyl esters,
  carcinogenicity and chemical reactivity, 59
GSH-S-transferases, see Glutathione S-epoxide
  transferase; Glutathione S-transferase-1,1
Guanidine, N-ethyl-N'-nitro N-nitroso-,
  direct-acting carcinogen, 9
—, N-methyl-N'-nitro-N-nitroso-,
  direct-acting carcinogen, 9
  DNA-repair and, 68
  tumour promotion of a subthreshold dose,
    102, 104
  methyldiazonium ions derived from, 24–25
  inhibition by reaction with nucleophiles, 94
  metabolic inhibitors and, 89–90
  reaction with DNA, 54–55
Guanine, O^6-alkyl-,
  in carcinogenesis,
    DNA-repair amd, 68–71
    DNA-synthesis and, 73–75
—, O^6-ethyl-,
  in DNA,
    and ethylating carcinogens, 54–55
—, O^6-methyl-,
  in DNA,
    and methylating carcinogens, 54–55

Hepatocarcinogenesis, 6–7, 15, 23, 37–38, 90,
  105–106, 108

132 Index

Hydrazine, 1,1-dimethyl-,
  methyldiazonium ions derived from a cyclic mechanism, 26–27
—, 1,2-dimethyl-,
  methyldiazonium ions derived from a cyclic mechanism, 26–27
  prevention of tumorigenesis with disulphiram, 88–89
  tissue-specific carcinogen, 15
Hydroxylamine, N-acetyl-2-fluorenyl-,
  metabolite of 2-AAF, 17–18
    reaction with DNA, 47–49
    tautomerism and activation, 20
—, N-acetyl-N-4-stilbenyl-,
  reaction with nucleic acids, 49–52
—, N-(4-biphenyl)-, 17, 18
  transport form, 21
—, N-(1-naphthyl)-,
  carcinogen from 1-naphthylamine, 17
  reaction with nucleic acids, carcinogenesis and, 50, 53
—, N-(2-naphthyl)-,
  carcinogen from 2-naphthylamine, 17–18
  transport form, 20–21

Inhibitors,
  of tumour induction,
    as metabolic inducers and inhibitors, 86–95
Isothiocyanate, benzyl-,
  as inhibitor of polycyclic aromatic hydrocarbon tumours, 88
—, phenethyl-,
  inhibitor of polycyclic aromatic hydrocarbon tumours, 88
—, phenyl-,
  inhibitor of polycyclic aromatic hydrocarbon tumours, 88

Ligandin, *see* Glutathione S-transferase-1,1

MMS, *see* Methyl methane sulphonate
MNNG, *see* Guanidine, N-methyl-N'-nitro-N-nitroso-
MNU, *see* Urea, N-methyl-N-nitroso-
MPT, *see* Triazene, 3-methyl-1-phenyl-
Metals,
  in human cancer, 4
  mechanism of carcinogenic action, 9–10, 29
    DNA-synthesis and, 76–77
    effect on RNA synthesis, 81
    reaction with DNA, 56
Methacrylic acid, methyl ester,
  generation of parent acid and its intermediary metabolism, 39–41
    possible spill-over model, 39
Methyl methane sulphonate,
  direct-acting carcinogen, 9

Methylation,
  via methyldiazonium ions, 24–29, 34–35
  of purine and pyrimidine bases in DNA, 54–55
Methyldiazonium ions,
  as methylating carcinogens, 24–29
Millers' electrophilic theory, 9
Miscoding,
  in DNA synthesis,
    aflatoxin B_1 and, 78
    alkylating carcinogens and, 73–76
    aromatic amines and, 79
    metals and, 76–77
    vinyl chloride-derived chloroacetaldehyde and, 77–78
Mutagenicity,
  correlation between miscoding in DNA and, 76–78, 124–125
  data, 16, 23–24, 36–39, 59, 68, 88
  theory, 7–8, 113–115

1-Naphthylamine,
  reactive metabolite, 17–18
  reaction with nucleic acids, carcinogenesis and, 50, 53
—, N-deoxyguanosin-O^6-yl-,
  from DNA and 1-naphthylamine, carcinogenesis and, 50, 53
—, 2-deoxyguanosin-O^6-yl-,
  from DNA and 1-napthylamine carcinogenesis and, 50, 53
2-Naphthylamine,
  industrial cancer, 2–3
  reaction with nucleic acids, *see* 1-Naphthylamine
  reactive metabolite, 17–18
  transport form and carcinogenicity, 8, 15–16, 20–21
Nickel,
  carcinogenesis, 4
  mutagenicity, 29
Nitrosamine, N-n-butyl-N-(4-hydroxybutyl)-,
  as alkylating carcinogen,
    disulphiram inhibition of carcinogenesis, 89
—, N,N-diethyl-,
  as ethylating carcinogen,
    effect of substances on tumour induction by, 86, 90–91
    effect on synthesis of inter-related macromolecules, 80
    mechanism of action, 9–10, 24–26, 54–55
    mutagenicity, 16
    tumour promotion of, 104
—, N,N-dimethyl-,
  as methylating carcinogen,
    DNA-repair of, 68–71
    effect of substances in tumour induction by, 90, 92, 94–95
    effect of synthesis of inter-related macromolecules, 80–82

Nitrosamine, N,N-dimethyl- (cont.)
  as methylating carcinogen (cont.)
    mechanism of action, 9–10, 24–26, 54–55
    miscoding in DNA by, 73–76
    mutagenicity, 16
    tumour promotion of, 102
No effect level,
  in carcinogenicity testing, 69–70
Nucleic acid synthesis,
  miscoding in,
    aflatoxin B_1 and, 78–79
    alkylating carcinogens and, 73–76
    N-fluoren-2-yl-acetamide and, 79
    metals and, 76–77
    vinyl chloride and, 77
Nucleosides,
  as nucleophiles against alkylating carcinogens, 94–95

'Oncogenes'/proto-oncogenes,
  viral proto-oncogenes,
    their mutation into 'oncogenes', 118–119
  activation of mammalian cell counterparts,
    by rearrangement of blocs of cellular sequences, 119–125

para-Red,
  as carcinogen, 23–24
Pearson's principle,
  of soft and hard acids and bases, carcinogenesis and, 10
Phenol, 2- and 3-$tert$-butyl-4-methoxy-,
  as inhibitor of polycyclic aromatic hydrocarbon, tumour induction, 87
Phenolic antioxidants,
  hindered,
    as inhibitors of tumour induction, 86–87
Phorbol-esters,
  as promoters of tumour induction in the skin system, 101–102
  as promoters of tumours in other tissues, 102
  their separation (from croton oil) and preparation, 102–103
  —, 12-O-tetradecanoyl-13-acetate(TPA),
    mechanism of tumour promotion in the skin, 107–109
Platinum(II), cis-diaminodichloro-,
  as mutagen,
    mechanism of action, 56
Polycyclic aromatic hydrocarbons,
  as human and animal carcinogens, 3–5
  inhibition of tumours, 87–88
  promotion of tumours, 101–102
  reaction with DNA, 61–64
    persistence of products in DNA, 72
  reactive epoxide metabolites, 31–33
Ponceau 3R,
  as carcinogen, 22–23

Product analysis,
  significance of products (nucleoside analogues, adducts) formed in DNA,
    from aflatoxin B_1, 78–79
    alkylating agents, 68–71, 73–76
    aromatic amines and their derivatives, 79
    metals, 76–77
    polycyclic aromatic hydrocarbons, 72
    vinyl chloride, 72, 77
  significance of products formed in RNA etc.,
    from alkylating agents, 79–82
    metals, 81

Retinoids,
  as inhibitors of tumour induction, 90
Retro- (or RNA-) viruses, see Tumour viruses
Riboflavin,
  as cofactor of azo-reductase,
    special inhibitor of tumour induction, 90–91

Saccharin,
  as promoter of bladder tumours, 104–105
Safrole,
  carcinogenicity,
    mechanism, 35–36
    reaction with DNA, 9, 63–64
Selenium,
  as inhibitor of tumour induction of amino-azo dyes, 91
Stilbene, N-acetoxy-4-acetamido-,
  reaction with adenosine, 50–51
    cytidine, 48–50
    guanosine, 50–52

TCE, see Ethylene, 1,1,2-trichloro-
Thiodiglycolic acid,
  metabolite of vinyl chloride, 30
    vinylidene chloride, 93
Thymine, O^4-alkyl-,
  in carcinogenesis,
    DNA-synthesis and, 73–76
  —, O^4-methyl-,
    DNA-synthesis and, 73–76
Tissue specificity,
  factors involved, 14–16, 36–41, 68–71, 89–92
o-Tolidine,
  mutagen from Trypan Blue, 22–23
Toluene, 4-hydroxy3,5-di-$tert$-butyl-,
  as inhibitor of polycyclic aromatic hydrocarbon tumour induction, 85–87
Transfection (or gene-transfer) focus assay, 119–121
Triazene,3,3-dimethyl-1-phenyl-,
  as methylating carcinogen,
    DNA-repair and, 68–71
    mechanism of action, 54–55

134 *Index*

Triazene, (*cont.*)
—,3,3-dimethyl-1-(2,4,6-trichlorophenyl)-,
　methyldiazonium ions derived from cyclic
　　mechanism, 28–29
　DNA-repair and, 68–71
　transport form of, 28–29
—, 3-methyl-1-phenyl-,
　as methylating carcinogen, 25–26, 28–29, 54–55
5-(1-Triazeno)imidazole-4-carboxamide, 3,3-dimethyl-,
　as cancer chemotherapeutic agent,
　transport form of, 28–29
Trypan Blue,
　as carcinogen, 22–23
Tumour viruses, 115–117
　retro- (or RNA-) viruses, 118–119
　viral proto-oncogenes,
　　their mutation into 'oncogenes', 118–119, 121

UDP-glucuronyl transferase,
　activities during inhibition of tumour induction, 86–87, 89

Urea, *N*-ethyl-*N*-nitroso-,
　as ethylating carcinogen, 9
　　DNA-repair and, 68–71
　ethyldiazonium ions derived from, 24–26
　　reaction with DNA, 54–55
—, *N*-hydroxy-,
　protection against Me-N$_2^+$ tumours, 94–95
—, *N*-methyl-*N*-nitroso-,
　as methylating carcinogen, 9
　　DNA-repair and, 68–71
　　tumour promotion of subthreshold dose, 104
　methyldiazonium ions derived from, 24–26
　　metabolic inhibitors and, 89–90
　　reaction with DNA, 54–55

Vinyl chloride,
　carcinogenesis, 7, 14, 37–38
　　mechanism and DNA interaction, 56–58, 72, 77–78, 124
　metabolites, 30
　mutagenicity, 16, 77–78
Vinylidene chloride,
　metabolism, 93–94